OVARIAN CANCER
PATIENT ADVOCATE

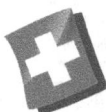

HealthScouter
WWW.HEALTHSCOUTER.COM

HealthScouter.com - Equity Press
5055 Canyon Crest Drive
Riverside, California 92507

www.healthscouter.com

Purchasing this book entitles you to free updates at www.healthscouter.com/OvarianCancer

Edited By: Katrina Robinson

Includes Ovarian Cancer from Wikipedia http://en.wikipedia.org/wiki/Ovarian_cancer

HealthScouter Ovarian Cancer Patient Advocate: Ovarian Cancer Symptoms and Signs of Ovarian Cancer (HealthScouter Ovarian Cancer)

ISBN 978-1-60332-108-2

Important

NEVER DISREGARD PROFESSIONAL MEDICAL ADVICE, OR DELAY SEEKING IT, BECAUSE OF SOMETHING YOU HAVE READ IN THIS BOOK. ALWAYS SEEK PROFESSIONAL MEDICAL ADVICE BEFORE ACTING UPON INFORMATION READ IN THIS BOOK.

HealthScouter and Equity Press do not provide medical advice. The contents of this book are for informational purposes only and are not intended to substitute for professional medical advice, diagnosis or treatment. Always seek advice from a qualified physician or health care professional about any medical concern, and do not disregard professional medical advice because of anything you may read in this book or on a HealthScouter Web site. The views of individuals quoted in this book are not necessarily those of HealthScouter or Equity Press.

While this book is intended to be a medium for the exchange of information and ideas, it is not meant in any way to be a substitute for sound medical advice; neither should it be viewed as a trusted source of such advice. The views expressed in these messages are not those of any qualified medical association, and the publisher is not responsible for the validity of the information communicated herein or for consequences that may arise from acting upon this information. The publisher is not responsible for any content found in the book that may be deemed offensive, inappropriate, inaccurate or medically unsound. The information you find here is only for the purpose of discussion and should not be the basis for any medical decision. The content is not intended to be a substitute for professional medical advice, diagnosis or treatment.

The information presented is not to be considered complete, nor does it contain all medical resource information that may be relevant, and therefore it is not intended to be a substitute for seeking medical treatment and/or appropriate care.

By reading this book and parts of the Web site, you agree under all circumstances to hold harmless, and to refrain from seeking remedy from, the owners of this book. The publisher shall disclaim all liability to you for damages, costs or expenses, including legal and medical fees, related to your reliance on anything derived from this book or Web site or its contents. Furthermore, Equity Press assumes no liability for any and all claims arising out of the said use, regardless of the cause, effects, or fault.

Equity Press and HealthScouter do not endorse any company or product, and listing on the HealthScouter Web site is not linked to corporate sponsorship. We do not make a claim to being comprehensive or up to date. If you would like to recommend information to include in this book, please contact us – we would be very happy to hear from you.

Purchasing this book entitles you to free updates as they are available. Please register your book at www.healthscouter.com

TABLE OF CONTENTS

INTRODUCTION AND MOTIVATION

Dear Reader,

I like to think of myself as a polite, well-reasoned person. I rarely speak out or complain. When a waitress spills something on me, or if my meal is cold—or if I'm overcharged—I generally try to be as polite as possible. I don't like to make very many waves. I often secretly hope that the manager will hear about my predicament and come out and offer me a free meal, or something similar. I generally hope that my polite and respectful demeanor pays off. And it does happen from time to time. You know, I think many people are brought up to believe that this is just good manners. It's how you're supposed to behave. And if you knew me personally, I think you'd agree that I'm generally pretty reserved. Of course my wife may raise an objection or two (!), but I really believe that it's important to treat others as you would like to be treated. We're talking about the golden rule here—it works well and it applies to almost every life circumstance.

But I have to admit that when it comes to my health, or the health of someone I care about—all bets are off. I want to know what's going on—when, why, where, and how. And I make these feelings known. I tend to get downright assertive. It's just something I feel very strongly about. And I feel that when you are in a hospital, or if you're brushing up against the healthcare system, that you should feel the same way. It's unfamiliar turf, and the professionals who work in this system often take advantage of their positions. They may use some jargon to hide the whole truth— or they may say something without checking to make sure you understand completely. They may present the options that are best for them, perhaps the most profitable or convenient. Now I'm not saying this goes on everywhere. There are many professionals in the business of health who go out of their way to make sure you have the best care. And I'm not suggesting that you should become a bully, or purposefully annoying—absolutely not. But I am suggesting that I think it's OK for you to step outside of your typical comfort zone, and put on your patient advocate hat. Because you, the patient or patient advocate, care the most about your care—not the medical system or healthcare providers.

HealthScouter was created to help patients become better advocates for their own medical care. Because when it comes to your healthcare, the stakes are high. There are none higher. And healthcare is one area where consumers (us, the sick people) are notoriously unaware of their options. And that's why I'm publishing these books. To help you understand your options, and to help you get the best care possible. I want to help you become a better advocate for yourself and for your loved ones.

It's my sincere hope that you can take this book with you to the hospital, to be read in the waiting room or by the bedside—and when you see a relevant patient comment you can use this book to ask questions of your health care providers. My advice: Ask lots of questions! Providers are busy people who generally go about their business with little questioning, delivering care as they see fit—making quick decisions—and again, nobody is going to care as much about your health as you. So now, more than ever, you need tools at your disposal to get the best care possible. One of the tools at your disposal is this HealthScouter book and the material within. You need to be armed with questions, and you need to ask questions all of the time. And so the difficult part is now to understand the right questions to ask.

That brings me to an explanation of how these books are structured. HealthScouter books include a number of what we call patient comments. These patient comments are summaries of what people have experienced. They're first hand accounts of what you may expect. These experiences effectively help you "catch up," and understand what outcomes are possible. They expose you to the treatments are available, and provide insight as to potential outcomes. They help you understand what other people are doing. So if you find yourself stuck feeling like you're receiving substandard medical care—or if you need a push to broach the subject, you can take this book to your provider and say, "Hey, I read here that another patient had this treatment—is that an option for me? If not, Why?" I believe that other peoples' experience is the most valuable way for you to formulate and build a list of good questions for your healthcare providers.

That notion is at the core of the HealthScouter philosophy.

So HealthScouter, by providing patient comments about a particular medical condition, will help expose you to what other people have experienced about a particular medical problem. If you know what other people have experienced, you can better understand what your options are. You'll be better informed and you'll have some questions to ask—it'll be like you've had access to dozens of other people who have gone through the same thing you're going through. And so armed, maybe you'll be able to move through your condition and get back on the road to health, and maybe you'll be able to do this with more grace than I have. And that is my sincere wish.

It's also my wish that perhaps when a doctor or nurse sees this little blue book, that they'll think twice about the care they're about to provide—knowing that the owner is a little bit better prepared, a little bit better armed—and yes, maybe even downright assertive.

I hope this book helps.

Yours truly,

Jim Stewart

San Diego, California

HOW TO USE THIS BOOK

The purpose of HealthScouter is to help you understand your medical condition as quickly and easily as possible. We believe this can best be accomplished by reading about other people and their experiences negotiating their health and care. We try to leave out complicated medical jargon. And we've spent a considerable amount of time structuring this book so that it's easy to use. It's important to know that this is not the sort of book you read from beginning to end. Of course you may do so, but this book is more meaningful if you flip through quickly and scan for applicable material. Again, it's all about the patient commentary: The darkly shaded comments ▬ indicate one patient initiating a new discussion, and the light or clear comments ▭ are other comments associated with that same condition. So you should begin by looking for information from other patients who are experiencing the same aspect of the same medical condition that you studying. You can do this quickly by scanning through the book, focusing on the dark shaded comment boxes. By scanning the patient comments you'll find information about various aspects of a condition, all grouped together, in an easy-to-read format. In this way you can immediately begin reading about other patients and their experiences with your particular medical condition – and you can benefit immediately from their experiences.

INTRODUCTION TO OVARIAN CANCER

Ovarian cancer is a cancerous growth arising from different parts of the ovary.

The most common form of ovarian cancer (≥80%) arises from the outer lining (epithelium) of the ovary.[1] Other forms arise from the egg cells (germ cell tumor).

In 2004, 25,580 new cases were diagnosed and 16,090 women died of ovarian cancer. The risk increases with age and decreases with pregnancy. Lifetime risk is about 1.6%, but women with affected first-degree relatives have a 5% risk. Women with a mutated BRCA1 or BRCA2 gene have a 25% risk.[2] Ovarian cancer is the fifth leading cause of death from cancer in women and the leading cause of death from gynecological cancer.[3]

10-year relative survival ranges from 84.1% in stage IA to 10.4% in stage IIIC.[4]

Ovarian cancer causes non-specific symptoms, which contribute to diagnostic delay, resulting in a late stage and a poor prognosis.[5] Most women with ovarian cancer report one or more symptoms such as abdominal pain or discomfort, an abdominal mass, bloating, back pain, urinary urgency, constipation, tiredness and a range of other non-specific symptoms, as well as more specific symptoms such as pelvic pain, abnormal vaginal bleeding or involuntary weight loss.[6][7][8] There can be a build-up of fluid in the abdominal cavity (this is called ascites).

An abnormal physical examination (including a pelvic examination), a blood test (for CA-125, more specifically) or medical imaging studies can provide evidence leading to an ovarian cancer diagnosis. The diagnosis can be confirmed with a surgical procedure (open or keyhole surgery) to inspect the abdominal cavity, take biopsies (tissue samples for microscopic analysis) and look for cancer cells in the abdominal fluid. Treatment usually involves chemotherapy and surgery, and sometimes radiotherapy.[9]

In most cases, the cause of ovarian cancer remains unknown. Older women, and in those who have a first or second degree relative with the disease, have an increased risk. Hereditary forms of ovarian cancer can be caused by mutations in specific genes (most notably BRCA1 and BRCA2, but also in genes for hereditary nonpolyposis colorectal cancer). Infertile women and those with a condition called endometriosis, those who have never been pregnant and those who use postmenopausal estrogen replacement therapy are at increased risk. Use of oral contraceptive pills is a protective factor. The risk is also lower in women who have had their uterine tubes blocked surgically (tubal ligation).[10][11]

I went to my gynecologist for my annual exam Thursday. All has been going well with me EXCEPT there has been two occasions where I have had a full bloated feeling. Keep in mind this has only happened twice in almost two years so I contributed this to just something going on with my gastrointestinal tract and it clears up in about five days. My only other problem has been some pain in the ovary area a few times. Again this may only happen once or twice a year and has occurred over a period of years. I happened to mention it to my doctor since it has recently happened on my left side and normally it is always on my right. I am 59 and post menopausal. He has scheduled me for a transvaginal ultrasound (or sonogram) to just "make sure" that all is okay. I am adopted so there is no medical history and he says that ovarian cancer has a tendency to be genetic.

Any words of wisdom?

If your symptoms have been going on for two years and haven't increased in severity or frequency, there's probably little to worry about. Ovarian cancer usually advances very quickly.

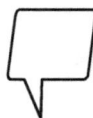

As far as I know, the bloated feeling doesn't go away when you have ovarian cancer and the cancer advances quickly. A friend of mine, sadly, has ovarian cancer and her belly got bigger and bigger. As far as the pain in the ovaries, I've had that off and on for a long time. I have ovarian cysts which are painful.

EPIDEMIOLOGY

The exact cause is usually unknown. The disease is more common in industrialized nations, with the exception of Japan. In the United States, females have a 1.4% to 2.5% (1 out of 40–60 women) lifetime chance of developing ovarian cancer. Older women are at highest risk. More than half of the deaths from ovarian cancer occur in women between 55 and 74 years of age and approximately one quarter of ovarian cancer deaths occur in women between 35 and 54 years of age.

The risk of developing ovarian cancer appears to be affected by several factors. The more children a woman has, the lower her risk of ovarian cancer. Early age at first pregnancy, older age of final pregnancy and the use of low dose hormonal contraception have also been shown to have a protective effect. Ovarian cancer is reduced in women after tubal ligation.

The relationship between use of oral contraceptives and ovarian cancer was shown in a summary of results of 45 case-control and prospective studies. Cumulatively these studies show a protective effect for ovarian cancers. Women who used oral contraceptives for 10 years had about a 60% reduction in risk of ovarian cancer (risk ratio .42 with statistical significant confidence intervals given the large study size, not unexpected). This means that if 250 women took oral contraceptives for 10 years, one ovarian cancer would be prevented. This is by far the largest epidemiological study to date on this subject (45 studies, over 20,000 women with ovarian cancer and about 80,000 controls).[12]

The link to the use of fertility medication, such as Clomiphene citrate, has been controversial. An analysis in 1991 raised the possibility that use of drugs may increase the risk of ovarian cancer. Several cohort studies and case-control studies have been conducted since then without demonstrating conclusive evidence for such a link.[13] It will remain a complex topic to study as the infertile population differs in parity from the "normal" population.

There is good evidence that in some women genetic factors are important. Carriers of certain mutations of the BRCA1 or the BRCA2 gene are notably at risk. The BRCA1 and BRCA2 genes account for 5%–13% of ovarian cancers[14] and certain populations (e.g. Ashkenazi Jewish women) are at a higher risk of both breast cancer and ovarian cancer, often at an earlier age than the general population. Patients with a personal history of breast cancer or a family history of breast and/or ovarian cancer, especially if diagnosed at a young age, may have an elevated risk.

A strong family history of uterine cancer, colon cancer, or other gastrointestinal cancers may indicate the presence of a syndrome known as hereditary nonpolyposis colorectal cancer (HNPCC, also known as Lynch II syndrome), which confers a higher risk for developing ovarian cancer. Patients with strong genetic risk for ovarian cancer may consider the use of prophylactic, i.e. preventative, oophorectomy after completion of childbearing.

A Swedish study, which followed more than 61,000 women for 13 years, has found a significant link between milk consumption and ovarian cancer. According to the BBC, "[Researchers] found that milk had the strongest link with ovarian cancer—those women who drank two or more glasses a day were at double the risk of those who did not consume it at all, or only in small amounts." [15] Recent studies have shown that women in sunnier countries have a lower rate of ovarian cancer, which may have some kind of connection with exposure to Vitamin D.

Other factors that have been investigated, such as talc use, asbestos exposure, high dietary fat content, and childhood mumps infection, are controversial and have not been definitively proven.

I have been having pain and bloating in my abdomen. I am also having constipation and gas. I have had a hysterectomy and both ovaries have been removed. I didn't think cancer was possible but an email told me it was. So if anyone knows the symptoms for either ovarian or peritoneal cancer or a reason for symptoms I am having please let me know. I have had breast cancer in the past and hope that these symptoms are just irritable bowel syndrome.

The symptoms you're having may have nothing to do with cancer. First place I would start is with a good gastroenterologist. They'd probably want to do either a GI series or a colonoscopy. Gas and bloating can be caused by diverticulosis, which are pockets in the intestines. They trap gas and some of the food you eat, so the food stays around longer for the intestinal bacteria to work on. Sometimes a change in diet can help. Also, diverticulosis is not in itself a problem, but if the pockets get infected (which is then called diverticulitis), it's very dangerous.

It's also possible you could have Irritable Bowel Syndrome, Infectious Bowel Disease, or other bowel problems.

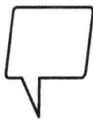

I had all those symptoms for years and I just recently got diagnosed with stage 3 ovarian cancer. I had a complete hysterectomy and a part of my bowel removed. I don't want to scare you but you need to have a ca-125 blood test and an ultrasound.

ALCOHOL

A pooled analysis of ten prospective cohort studies conducted in a number of countries and including 529,638 women found that neither total alcohol consumption nor alcohol from drinking beer, wine or spirits was associated with ovarian cancer risk."[16] The results of a case-control study in the region of Milan, Italy, "suggests that relatively elevated alcohol intake (of the order of 40 g per day or more) may cause a modest increase of epithelial ovarian cancer risk"[17]. "Associations were also found between alcohol consumption and cancers of the ovary and prostate, but only for 50 g and 100 g a day."[18] "Statistically significant increases in risk also existed for cancers of the stomach, colon, rectum, liver, female breast, and ovaries."[19]

CLASSIFICATION

Ovarian cancer is classified according to the histology of the tumor, obtained in a pathology report. Histology dictates many aspects of clinical treatment, management, and prognosis.

• Surface epithelial-stromal tumor, also known as ovarian epithelial carcinoma, is the most common type of ovarian cancer. It includes serous tumor, endometrioid tumor and mucinous cystadenocarcinoma.

• Sex cord-stromal tumor, including estrogen-producing granulosa cell tumor and virilizing Sertoli-Leydig cell tumor or arrhenoblastoma, accounts for 8% of ovarian cancers.

• Germ cell tumor accounts for approximately 30% of ovarian tumors but only 5% of ovarian cancers, because most germ cell tumors are teratomas and most teratomas are benign. Germ cell tumor tends to occur in young women and girls. The prognosis depends on the specific histology of germ cell tumor, but overall is favorable.

• Mixed tumors, containing elements of more than one of the above classes of tumor histology.

Ovarian cancer can also be a secondary cancer, the result of metastasis from a primary cancer elsewhere in the body. Common primary cancers are breast cancer and gastrointestinal cancer (in which case the ovarian cancer is a Krukenberg cancer). Surface epithelial-stromal tumor can originate in the peritoneum (the lining of the abdominal cavity), in which case the ovarian cancer is secondary to primary peritoneal cancer, but treatment is basically the same as for primary surface epithelial-stromal tumor involving the peritoneum.

> *A few months ago I was diagnosed with polycystic ovary disease. They sent me for an ultrasound and it turns out I have a 14cm cyst with, apparently, something about the echo readings that required further testing. So I had an abdominal CT scan done, and then a pelvic exam by my gynecologist. I just got the results back from the CT scan and they said the "pelvic mass" required further evaluation, so they've scheduled me for an MRI. I'm supposed to have a laparatomy next month.*
>
> *I'm getting a little nervous about all of this... to have gone from one month thinking everything was fine in the world to learning I have polycystic ovary disease and could potentially*

have all kinds of problems, to finding out I have this enormous cyst, then to have all these tests, including all kinds of blood tests. I'm just wondering what all these tests could mean... if anyone has any ideas? Why would they need an ultrasound and a CT and an MRI?

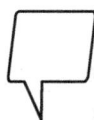

Have they also ordered a blood test called the CA-125 ? This is a test that looks for a specific cancer antigen that is usually present in high numbers when ovarian cancer is present. 35 and under is normal. Unfortunately, pre-menopausal women have a greater chance of having either a false positive (where you score high and there is no cancer) or a false negative (where you score normal and there is stage 1 ovarian cancer) than post menopausal women. However, this can nevertheless be a source of additional information and I am rather surprised that your doctors have not requested this test.

Usually the ultrasound is the gold standard for ovarian cysts and the only reason I can think of to do the MRI would be to check out the rest of that area and be sure there is nothing that the ultrasound may have missed. I am not sure why they would call for both a CT scan AND an MRI, so perhaps you should ask your doctor about this.

If cancer is at all suspected, you absolutely NEED to have this surgery done by a gynecological oncologist. These gynecologists are specially trained in this field and should cancer be present, they can take the proper precautions during the surgery.

Even very large cysts such as yours are quite common, even in younger women. The likelihood that it is something dangerous is extremely small.

SYMPTOMS

Two case-control studies, both subject to results being inflated by spectrum bias, have been reported. The first found that women with ovarian cancer had symptoms of increased abdominal size, bloating, urge to pass urine and pelvic pain.[8] The smaller, second study found that women with ovarian cancer had pelvic/abdominal pain, increased abdominal size/bloating, and difficulty eating/feeling full.[21] The latter study created a symptom index that was considered positive if any of the six symptoms "occurred under 12 times per month but were present for over one year". They reported a sensitivity of 57% for early-stage disease and specificity 87% to 90%.

I'm a 57-year-old woman who has had an adnexal cyst for as long as I can remember. For the past 10 years I have had the cyst monitored by ultrasound every six months. It has always shown to be fluid filled around 2.5 cm. My last ultrasound was last month, and I was shocked to find that things have changed for the worse. It is now slightly larger at 3 cm but also now has a solid component protruding into the cyst with 4 mm echogenic focus. Unfortunately, the technologist did not access for Doppler vascularity. Given my age and the results, I am fully prepared for the finding to be ovarian cancer. My doctor has referred me to a gynecologist. It's been three weeks since the referral and I'm way down on the waiting list and still do not know when my initial appointment will be. My concern is that I read on the internet that ovarian cancer is very fast growing and can go from stage 1 to stage 4 within a year. Is this true?

I was in exactly your situation over the past years. In 2007 they discovered an ovarian simple cyst which was about 7 cm. At that time, all the doctors said that it was a normal follicular cyst but at my follow up ultrasound it had grown just slightly to around 7.5 cm. Like you, I had follow-up ultrasounds every six months and it grew in increments of .3 to .5 cm at a time. Then at one point my cyst developed a very small solid part of a few mms and this made me extremely nervous. My gynecologist at that time told me that a few mm was nothing to worry about and the radiologist said that this sometimes happens with cysts that have been there for a long time. Finally, this past February I went for an ultrasound and the cyst was almost 9 cm. The radiologist compared this result to all of my previous results and said that although the cyst did not look dangerous, it was taking up space and he left it up to the treating physician to decide whether or not to remove it. My gynecologist told me that perhaps it was time, since I did not want to have a more complicated surgery to remove it later on. I had surgery this past April 28th and as suspected, it was a benign serous cyst.

Having been in your shoes, here is what I would recommend to you:

1. Get a copy of the radiology report and read it.

2. Contact your general practitioner and see if he or she can send you for a CA-125 test. This is a simple blood test that checks for a cancer antigen that is normally present in high numbers when ovarian cancer is present

3. Ask your friends and family for gynecologist recommendations and start phoning around to see if anyone can take you sooner.

Ovarian Cancer Symptoms Consensus Statement

In 2007, the Gynecologic Cancer Foundation, Society of Gynecologic Oncologists and American Cancer

Society originated the following consensus statement regarding the symptoms of ovarian cancer.[22]

Ovarian cancer is called a "silent killer" because symptoms were not thought to develop until the disease had advanced and the chance of cure or remission poor. However, the following symptoms are much more likely to occur in women with ovarian cancer than women in the general population. These symptoms include:

• Bloating

• Pelvic or abdominal pain

• Pain in the back or legs

• Diarrhea, gas, nausea, constipation, indigestion

• Difficulty eating or feeling full quickly

• Urinary symptoms (urgency or frequency)

• Pain during sex

• Abnormal vaginal bleeding

• Trouble breathing

Women with ovarian cancer report that symptoms are persistent and represent a change from normal for their bodies. The frequency and/or number of such symptoms are key factors in the diagnosis of ovarian cancer. Several studies show that even early stage ovarian cancer can produce these symptoms. Women who have these symptoms almost daily for more than a few weeks should see their doctor, preferably a gynecologist. Prompt medical evaluation may lead to detection at the earliest possible stage of the disease. Early stage diagnosis is associated with an improved prognosis.

Several other symptoms have been commonly reported by women with ovarian cancer. These symptoms include fatigue, indigestion, back pain, pain with intercourse, constipation and menstrual irregularities. However, these other symptoms are not as useful in identifying ovarian cancer because they are also found in equal frequency in women in the general population who do not have ovarian cancer.

I have noticed this month a pain on the right side of my body from the bottom of my appendectomy scar to my pubic bone. I am 43 and very likely in perimenopause due to the symptoms I have been experiencing for the last year. I have noticed that I am more prone to urinary irritabilities over the last year. My question is where is the pain from an ovarian cyst? The pain is not terribly bad; I have no abnormal bleeding, no bloating, no nausea. I have an appointment on Thursday with the gynecologist, but the thought flitters through my mind occasionally about the possibility of it being ovarian cancer. The only thing that "raises" my risk of ovarian cancer is my mom's breast cancer diagnosis. I don't know if anyone can give me any more info but if someone can I would appreciate it.

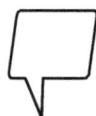

Why not ask your gynecologist to follow up on this with a pelvic ultrasound? This should uncover any problems with your ovaries. If they see anything and you are concerned about ovarian cancer, then you can always get the CA-125 blood test to see where you are (a score of 35 and under is considered normal for this cancer antigen). 43 is a tiny bit early to be going into peri-menopause, but not unusual.

DIAGNOSIS

Ovarian cancer at its early stages (I/II) is difficult to diagnose until it spreads and advances to later stages (III/IV). This is due to the fact that most of the common symptoms are non-specific.

When an ovarian malignancy is included in the list of diagnostic possibilities, a limited number of laboratory tests are indicated. A complete blood count (CBC) and serum electrolyte test should be obtained in all patients.

The serum BHCG level should be measured in any female in whom pregnancy is a possibility. In addition, serum alpha-fetoprotein (AFP) and lactate dehydrogenase (LDH) should be measured in young girls and adolescents with suspected ovarian tumors because the younger the patient, the greater the likelihood of a malignant germ cell tumor.

A blood test called CA-125 is useful in differential diagnosis and in follow up of the disease, but it by itself has not been shown to be an effective method to screen for early-stage ovarian cancer due to its unacceptable low sensitivity and specificity. However, this is the only available, widely-used marker currently.

Current research is looking at ways to combine tumor markers proteomics along with other indicators of disease (i.e. radiology and/or symptoms) to improve accuracy. The challenge in such an approach is that the very low population prevalence of ovarian cancer means that even testing with very high sensitivity and specificity will still lead to a number of false positive results (i.e. performing surgical procedures in which cancer is not found intra-operatively). However, the contributions of proteomics are still in the early stages and require further refining. Current studies on proteomics mark the beginning of a paradigm shift towards individually tailored therapy.

A pelvic examination and imaging including CT scan and trans-vaginal ultrasound are essential. Physical examination may reveal increased abdominal girth and/or ascites (fluid within the abdominal cavity). Pelvic examination may reveal an ovarian or abdominal mass. The pelvic examination can include a rectovaginal component for better palpation of the ovaries. For very young patients, magnetic resonance imaging may be preferred to rectal and vaginal examination.

To definitively diagnose ovarian cancer, a surgical procedure to take a look into the abdomen is required. This can be an open procedure (laparotomy, incision through the abdominal wall) or keyhole surgery (laparoscopy). During this procedure, suspicious areas will be removed and sent for microscopic analysis. Fluid from the abdominal cavity can also be analyzed for cancerous cells. If there is cancer, this procedure can also determine its spread (which is a form of tumor staging).

I've had a lot of the symptoms that go along with ovarian cancer and tomorrow I go in for an ultrasound. It's about to be "that time of the month" for me, so my question is, can they read an ultrasound clearly if I'm about due for my period? Also, could some of you share your symptoms?

It is fine as long as you don't have your period in full force. I had an ultrasound and I was at the very end of my period and spotting a little, which they told me was fine. My ultrasound results showed a fibroid in my uterus and a cyst on my ovary. It is my understanding that these things are common. It's good that you are going to get it checked out then you will know for sure what it is and how to handle it.

Screening

The goal of ovarian cancer screening is to detect ovarian cancer at stage I although it may be better to screen for low-volume.[23] Until 2009 routine screening could not be recommended because of poor specificity resulting in unnecessary surgery for false-positive screening results.[24] In 2009, however, Menon et al. reported from the UKCTOCS that utilizing multimodal screening, in essence first performing annual CA 125 testing, followed by ultrasound imaging on the secondary level, the positive predictive value was 35.1% for primary invasive epithelial ovarian and tubal carcinoma, making such screening feasible.[25] However, it remains to be seen if such screening is effective to reduce mortality.

I'm 40, a single mom, with four sons. Just over a month ago I noticed left sided groin pain, radiating into my hip and even down my leg. The pain is severely worsened upon sitting in the car or a straight chair. A week after the pain began, I had another skin biopsy on the shin of that leg and so I assumed it would be positive and the groin pain was the skin cancer having spread to the lymph node. The pain was so unbearable it was keeping me up at night, so I went to see my rheumatologist, thinking it

could be arthritis. She said no, and confirmed
there was lymph node swelling, advised heat
and prescribed pain relievers. The skin biopsy
came back as precancerous... but the groin
pain continued. I called my rheumatologist; she
advised going to see a lymphoma doctor. By this
time, I had noticed my abdomen looking bloated
even though I have lost some weight. And for
about a week I've had gas that seems completely
unrelated to what I've been eating.

I went in to see my gynecologist yesterday. My
period had just ended, and I'm not certain if the
pain is slightly better or if I'm getting used to
it or if because I take the pain pills. So, I really
don't want anything to be wrong, and now I'm
worried that I may have down played this to him.
He did the pelvic exam and when he touched my
left ovary, I screamed, bit my hand to keep from
kicking him, and literally cried, tears running
down my cheeks. He did an ultrasound and said
he didn't see anything. And the lymph nodes in
my groin are no longer swollen.

He suggested that I probably had a cyst, that
it ruptured on its own and that the pain is now
slowly starting to feel better and would resolve.

But since then, the pain has been worse. I've been telling myself it's because he manipulated my painful ovary.

If the pain continues, is it possible to request that he goes in and removes the ovary? Here is what I am looking for from women with experience: What were your symptoms? Was it difficult to diagnose? How would you advise me?

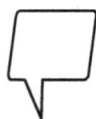

I seriously think that you need to find a doctor who will do the necessary tests in order to find out what is truly wrong with you. Ovarian cancer symptoms definitely include bloating and abdominal pain. Have you had an ultrasound to check for any abnormalities? Also, a CA-125 test is not a bad idea. This is a test that checks for a cancer antigen that is normally present with ovarian cancer. It is not always reliable but if the numbers are truly high (over 35) then it begs further testing (such as a CT scan). It is a blood test that can have results quickly.

Insist that they check for both ovarian (CA-125 blood test and abdomino-pelvic ultrasound), gastroenterology (colonoscopy or sigmoidoscopy) and bile duct issues (liver, pancreas, gall bladder).

Staging

Ovarian cancer staging is by the FIGO staging system and uses information obtained after surgery, which can include a total abdominal hysterectomy, removal of (usually) both ovaries and fallopian tubes, (usually) the omentum, and pelvic (peritoneal) washings for cytology. The AJCC stage is the same as the FIGO stage.

- Stage I - limited to one or both ovaries

  - IA - involves one ovary; capsule intact; no tumor on ovarian surface; no malignant cells in ascites or peritoneal washings

  - IB - involves both ovaries; capsule intact; no tumor on ovarian surface; negative washings

  - IC - tumor limited to ovaries with any of the following: capsule ruptured, tumor on ovarian surface, positive washings

- Stage II - pelvic extension or implants

  - IIA - extension or implants onto uterus or fallopian tube; negative washings

  - IIB - extension or implants onto other pelvic structures; negative washings

- IIC - pelvic extension or implants with positive peritoneal washings

- Stage III - microscopic peritoneal implants outside of the pelvis; or limited to the pelvis with extension to the small bowel or omentum

  - IIIA - microscopic peritoneal metastases beyond pelvis

  - IIIB - macroscopic peritoneal metastases beyond pelvis less than 2 cm in size

  - IIIC - peritoneal metastases beyond pelvis > 2 cm or lymph node metastases

- Stage IV - distant metastases to the liver or outside the peritoneal cavity

Para-aortic lymph node metastases are considered regional lymph nodes (Stage IIIC).

Today we found out my mom has ovarian cancer. They won't know the stage for another three days or so, but the doctor estimated it at 2c. He said the cancer is not on her liver or lungs. I'm so scared, what if he's estimating it too high? I'm not really sure what qualifies as a stage 2c and reading articles just confuses me.

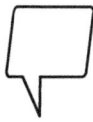

Ovarian cancer, and I think all cancers, are categorized in four stages. Each stage has three sub-stages, like stage 1A, 1B, 1C-2A, 2B, 2C, etc. A detailed description of the different stages follows.

> *Stage 1: The cancer is still contained within the ovary (or ovaries). Stage 1A: Cancer has developed in one ovary, and the tumor is confined to the inside of the ovary. There is no cancer on the outer surface of the ovary. Laboratory examination of washings from the abdomen and pelvis did not find any cancer cells. Stage 1B: Cancer has developed within both ovaries without any tumor on their outer surfaces. Laboratory examination of washings from the abdomen and pelvis did not find any cancer cells. Stage 1C: The cancer is present in one or both ovaries and one or more of the following are present: Cancer on the outer surface of at least one of the ovaries, in the case of cystic tumors (fluid-filled tumors), the capsule (outer wall of the tumor) has ruptured (burst), and/or laboratory examination found*

cancer cells in fluid or washings from the abdomen.

Stage 2: The cancer is in one or both ovaries and has involved other organs (such as the uterus, fallopian tubes, bladder, the sigmoid colon, or the rectum) within the pelvis. Stage 2A: The cancer has spread to or has actually invaded (grown into) the uterus or the fallopian tubes, or both. Laboratory examination of washings from the abdomen did not find any cancer cells. Stage 2B: The cancer has spread to other nearby pelvic organs such as the bladder, the sigmoid colon, or the rectum. Laboratory examination of fluid from the abdomen did not find any cancer cells. Stage 2C: The cancer has spread to pelvic organs as in stages IIA or IIB and laboratory examination of the washings from the abdomen found evidence of cancer cells.

Stage 3: The cancer involves one or both ovaries, and one or both of the following are present: (1) cancer has spread beyond the pelvis to the lining of the abdomen; (2) cancer has spread to lymph nodes.

Stage 3A: During the staging operation, the surgeon can see cancer involving the ovary or ovaries, but no cancer is grossly visible in the abdomen and the cancer has not spread to lymph nodes. However, when biopsies are checked under a microscope, tiny deposits of cancer are found in the lining of the upper abdomen. Stage 3B: There is cancer in one or both ovaries, and deposits of cancer large enough for the surgeon to see, but smaller than 2 cm (about 3/4 inch) across, are present in the abdomen. Cancer has not spread to the lymph nodes. Stage 3C: The cancer is in one or both ovaries, and one or both of the following are present: cancer has spread to lymph nodes, and/ or deposits of cancer larger than 2 cm (about 3/4 inch) across are seen in the abdomen (T3c, N0, M0).

Stage IV: This is the most advanced stage of ovarian cancer. In this stage the cancer has spread to the inside of the liver, the lungs, or other organs located outside of the peritoneal cavity. (The peritoneal cavity, or abdominal cavity is the area enclosed by the peritoneum, a. membrane that lines the inner abdomen and covers most of its organs.).

TREATMENT

Surgical treatment may be sufficient for malignant tumors that are well-differentiated and confined to the ovary. Addition of chemotherapy may be required for more aggressive tumors that are confined to the ovary. For patients with advanced disease a combination of surgical reduction with a combination chemotherapy regimen is standard. Borderline tumors, even following spread outside of the ovary, are managed well with surgery, and chemotherapy is not seen as useful.

Surgery is the preferred treatment and is frequently necessary to obtain a tissue specimen for differential diagnosis via its histology. Surgery performed by a specialist in gynecologic oncology usually results in an improved result. Improved survival is attributed to more accurate staging of the disease and a higher rate of aggressive surgical excision of tumor in the abdomen by gynecologic oncologists as opposed to general gynecologists and general surgeons.

The type of surgery depends upon how widespread the cancer is when diagnosed (the cancer stage), as well as the presumed type and grade of cancer. The surgeon may remove one (unilateral oophorectomy) or both ovaries (bilateral oophorectomy), the fallopian tubes (salpingectomy), and the uterus (hysterectomy). For some very early tumors (stage 1, low grade or low-risk disease), only the involved ovary and fallopian tube will be removed (called a "unilateral salpingo-oophorectomy," USO), especially in young females who wish to preserve their fertility.

In advanced malignancy, where complete resection is not feasible, as much tumor as possible is removed (debulking surgery). In cases where this type of surgery is successful (i.e. < 1 cm in diameter of tumor is left behind ["optimal debulking"]), the prognosis is improved compared to patients where large tumor masses (> 1 cm in diameter) are left behind. Minimally invasive surgical techniques may facilitate the safe removal of very large (greater than 10 cm) tumors with fewer complications of surgery.[26]

Chemotherapy has been a general standard of care for ovarian cancer for decades, although with highly variable protocols.[27] Chemotherapy is used after surgery to treat any residual disease, if appropriate. This depends on the histology of the tumor; some kinds of tumor (particularly teratoma) are not sensitive to chemotherapy. In some cases, there may be reason to perform chemotherapy first, followed by surgery.

For patients with stage IIIC epithelial ovarian adenocarcinomas who have undergone successful optimal debulking, a recent clinical trial demonstrated that median survival time is significantly longer for patient receiving intraperitoneal chemotherapy.[28] Patients in this clinical trial reported less compliance with intraperitoneal chemotherapy and fewer than half of the patients received all six cycles of intraperitoneal chemotherapy. Despite this high "drop-out" rate, the group as a whole (including the patients that didn't complete intraperitoneal chemotherapy treatment) survived longer on average than patients who received intravenous chemotherapy alone.

Some specialists believe the toxicities and other complications of intraperitoneal chemotherapy will be unnecessary with improved intravenous chemotherapy drugs currently being developed.

Although intraperitoneal chemotherapy has been recommended as a standard of care for the first-line treatment of ovarian cancer, the basis for this recommendation has been challenged.[29]

Radiation therapy is not effective for advanced stages because when vital organs are in the radiation field, a high dose cannot be safely delivered.

I am a 55-year-old woman who recently just had a complete hysterectomy and part of my bowel removed because I was diagnosed with stage 3 ovarian cancer, a rare form. I had my first chemotherapy and am starting a clinical trial on the 22nd of July. I am having a tough time eating and getting back on my feet after the first chemotherapy, which caused dizziness, leg pain, and now sores on my mouth. Just wondering if anyone had any of this.

I was 55 also when I was diagnosed with stage 3C ovarian cancer. I had a hysterectomy and part of my bowel removed, too. I was given Taxol and Carboplatin for six months every three weeks. I remember having muscle and leg pain. I have heard of people getting sores in their mouth. Chemotherapy can make you very fatigued, so try to get plenty of rest.

PROGNOSIS

Ovarian cancer usually has a poor prognosis. It is disproportionately deadly because it lacks any clear early detection or screening test, meaning that most cases are not diagnosed until they have reached advanced stages. More than 60% of patients presenting with this cancer already have stage III or stage IV cancer, when it has already spread beyond the ovaries. Ovarian cancers shed cells into the naturally occurring fluid within the abdominal cavity. These cells can implant on other abdominal (peritoneal) structures, included the uterus, urinary bladder, bowel and the lining of the bowel wall (omentum). These cells can begin forming new tumor growths before cancer is even suspected.

The five-year survival rate for all stages of ovarian cancer is 45.5%. For cases where a diagnosis is made early in the disease, when the cancer is still confined to the primary site, the five-year survival rate is 92.7%.[30]

Germ cell tumors of the ovary have a much better prognosis than other ovarian cancers, in part because they tend to grow rapidly to a very large size, hence they are detected sooner.

On 7th of January 2007, after the surgical intervention (hysterectomy and oophorectomy) of my wife, I was told that she had ovarian cancer stage 3C. They couldn't remove the entire tumor; a part of it had involved the pelvic artery and touched the bowel for. Chemotherapy was the next step, and at the end of it the CA125 decreased from about 500 to 8. After six months it raised up to 57 and they found that the tumor was back, in the same place. Another doctor, recommended by the first one, operated on my wife and said that all the tumor was removed this time. He suggested my wife follow the same protocol (paclitaxel/carboplatin) as the first one. After three cycles the CA125 dropped down to 6 but now, when chemo is finished (last cycle was three weeks ago), the CA is 12.

Is it possible that this time the treatment has not been efficient? Some doctors said that the second chemotherapy should be different. What should I expect now?

I was given six treatments of chemotherapy after my surgery over a six-month period. My CA125 level dropped a great deal. Then I had 12 treatments of what they called maintenance chemotherapy (taxol) over the next year. I have

*been done with chemotherapy for over a year and
I feel pretty good. I get my CA125 checked every
three months and a CT Scan every six months.*

*I think your wife's CA125 level of 12 is quite good;
I think anything under 30 is OK.*

Complications

• Spread of the cancer to other organs

• Progressive function loss of various organs

• Ascites (fluid in the abdomen)

• Intestinal obstructions

These cells can implant on other abdominal
(peritoneal) structures, including the uterus, urinary
bladder, bowel, lining of the bowel wall (omentum)
and, less frequently, to the lungs.

PREVENTION

There are a number of ways to reduce or eliminate the risk of ovarian cancer. Pregnancy before the age of 25 as well as breastfeeding provides some reduction in risk. Tubal ligation and hysterectomy reduce the risk and removal of both ovaries (bilateral oophorectomy) eliminates the risk. The use of oral contraceptives (birth control pills) for five years or more decreases the risk of ovarian cancer in later life by 50%.[31]

OVARIAN CYST

An ovarian cyst is any collection of fluid, surrounded by a very thin wall, within an ovary. Any ovarian follicle that is larger than about two centimeters is termed an ovarian cyst. An ovarian cyst can be as small as a pea, or larger than a cantaloupe.

Most ovarian cysts are functional in nature, and harmless (benign).[1] In the US, ovarian cysts are found in nearly all premenopausal women, and in up to 14.8% of postmenopausal women.

Ovarian cysts affect women of all ages. They occur most often, however, during a woman's childbearing years.

Some ovarian cysts cause problems, such as bleeding and pain. Surgery may be required to remove cysts larger than five centimeters in size.

Are ovarian cysts and cervical dysplasia linked? I was diagnosed with cervical dysplasia four months ago and was just recently diagnosed with ovarian cysts. Are these linked or is this just a coincidence?

Not that I know of. Cervical dysplasia can be caused by HPV. Women have ovarian cysts as part of their monthly cycles. There are other types of cysts that are not part of the cycle, but I don't understand a lot about them.

I had lower right side pain and an ultrasound revealed an ovarian cyst. I still had the pain when I went for my follow-up ultrasound, but it was gone. There was some residual fluid around the ovary. That was a month ago. I still had discomfort, which within the last few days has intensified like it was when I first told my doctor about the pain. My periods are regular.

At first my doctor told me that since I have fibromyalgia, it could just be that I feel the pain of the cyst more intensely than a non-fibromyalgia person would. But it's been a month since the ultrasound. Anyone have a similar experience?

It is normal for the ovary to create a small cyst when pushing the egg out of the ovary into the fallopian tube. It's also normal for it to go away after pushing that egg out. No doubt, the fibromyalgia plays into the pain. However, if it continues next month around ovulation, call your doctor again.

Types

Functional cysts

Some, called functional cysts, or simple cysts, are part of the normal process of menstruation. They have nothing to do with disease, and can be treated. There are three types: Graafian, Luteal, and Hemorrhagic. These types of cysts occur during ovulation. If the egg is not released, the ovary can fill up with fluid. Usually these types of cysts will go away after a few period cycles.

> *For the past six months I have been having severe pain on my lower back and pelvis area all the way down to my leg. At first I thought it was menstrual cramp and that it would go away, so I was taking pain medication every day and it seemed to get worse. I finally decided to go see a gynecologist and explain to him about the pain, which is unbearable. I couldn't sit, cough, sleep or do anything. When I went to the gynecologist, he told me it was nothing and quickly brushed me off and then I brought up the ovarian cyst and he said that it would go away. However, I've been having this pain for months.*

Last month I demanded an ultrasound and when the results came, he said the cyst was too small to cause this much pain, and that was it! He didn't recommend anything after that, so I decided to take some Tylenol, which worked for a few hours, but then the pain came back. Last week I went to the urgent care and the doctor gave me a CAT scan. The doctor said I have an 8cm ovarian cyst, but he brushed it off as not being serious. Should I be worried about this cyst? I am 26 and eventually want to have kids.

I was in a similar position about four years ago. I woke up one day with excruciating pain in my lower left buttock that extended around to my frontal pelvic area and down the inside of my leg. At first I took anti-inflammatory medication and the severe pain subsided. However, I began to notice that I still had a lot of pain in my front pelvic area and down my leg, and I noticed that the pain was more prevalent in the morning and during the night while I slept. Since I slept on my side, I thought it might be a mattress problem so I purchased a "topper" for my mattress made of memory foam, and this helped me immensely. My husband, who is in the medical field, also thought it might be a problem with my hip. At the time I *was significantly overweight and like you, I had just been diagnosed with a left ovarian cyst which was around 8 cm at the time.*

Despite the incredible coincidence, the cyst had NOTHING to do with my pain. When I lost 60 pounds, the pain decreased significantly, and when I added a daily morning walk to my routine, the pain almost went away completely. My cyst grew over time and I recently had it removed through surgery (along with my ovary and tube). I still have the occasional left hip problem, although it is still minor compared to four years ago.

Your cyst should be watched with ultrasounds to see if it goes away on its own, if it persists, changes or whatever. When I was first diagnosed with my 8 cm cyst, my general practitioner said that it was a totally normal functional cyst that we all get with ovulation. However, I was EXTREMELY skeptical (an 8 cm functional cyst?!) so I went to see a couple of different gynecologists to get opinions. None of them thought it was a functional cyst, although they all told me that it was harmless due to the fact that it was only fluid filled. With time this thing grew and began to experience slight changes so when it hit 9 cm, my gynecologist recommended I have it removed before it got bigger and needed a more serious surgery.

Graafian follicle cyst

One type of simple cyst, which is the most common type of ovarian cyst, is the graafian follicle cyst, or follicular cyst.

Corpus luteum cyst

Another is a corpus luteum cyst (which may rupture about the time of menstruation, and take up to three months to disappear entirely).

Hemorrhagic cyst

A third type of functional cyst, which is common, is a Hemorrhagic cyst, which is also called a blood cyst, hematocele, and hematocyst.[2] It occurs when a very small blood vessel in the wall of the cyst breaks, and the blood enters the cyst. Abdominal pain on one side of the body, often the right side, may be present. The bleeding may occur quickly, and rapidly stretch the covering of the ovary, causing pain. As the blood collects within the ovary, clots form which can be seen on a sonogram.[3][4] Occasionally hemorrhagic cysts can rupture, with blood entering the abdominal cavity. No blood is seen out of the vagina. If a cyst ruptures, it is usually very painful. Hemorrhagic cysts that rupture are less common. Most hemorrhagic cysts are self-limiting; some need surgical intervention. Even if a hemorrhagic cyst ruptures, in many cases it resolves without surgery. Patients who don't require surgery will experience pain for 4–10 days after, and may require several days rest. Studies have found that women on tetracycline antibiotics recover 25% earlier than the majority of patients, a surprising correlation found in 2004. Sometimes surgery is necessary,[5][6] such as a laparoscopy ("belly-button surgery" that uses small tools inserted through one or more tiny slits in the abdomen).[7]

I have been diagnosed with having a ~6 cm hemorrhagic septated ovarian cyst and a ~6 cm hemorrhagic simple ovarian cyst. Can they be treated via ultrasound guided aspiration (together with antibiotic therapy), or is surgery inevitable? Has anyone gone under such a procedure for such cysts?

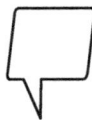

I believe that like simple cysts, hemorrhagic cysts can regress on their own, so your doctor may even recommend a simple follow-up ultrasound in a little while.

Your main issue is the septated cyst. Depending upon your health care physician, you may need to have this one removed and tested, just to be on the safe side. The most probable outcome is that they will want to do a laparoscopy to remove at least the septated cyst.

Antibiotics are not needed for cysts. Sometimes doctors put women on birth control pills because they believe that this rests the ovaries but it is now known that oral contraceptives are ineffective at either shrinking existing cysts or preventing new ones from growing. The latest generation of birth control pills interferes mostly with the hormone surge that occurs when an egg is released from a follicular cyst (i.e. ovulation) and not with the actual growth of functional cysts.

Endometrioid cyst

An endometrioma, endometrioid cyst, endometrial cyst, or chocolate cyst is caused by endometriosis, and formed when a tiny patch of endometrial tissue (the mucous membrane that makes up the inner layer of the uterine wall) bleeds, sloughs off, becomes transplanted, and grows and enlarges inside the ovaries.

I went to the emergency room a couple days ago and found out that I have an ovarian cyst

on my right ovary (it's 5.2 cm). My first question
is, how can I tell which one it is? I know you
may have to get a sonogram or something to tell
that but the doctor at the emergency room never
told me which one. My next question is could I
have ovarian cancer that they did not pick up?
I seem to have the symptoms of that. I've had
pressure and pain my lower abdomen as well
as my back, a bloated abdominal, nausea and
gas, tired more than usual, urinating more often,
and my periods have been different. Should I be
concerned?

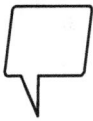

If they did an ultrasound at the emergency room,
which they should have in order to diagnose
your cyst, then you should be able to get a copy
of this. The report will say what type of cyst you
have. A simple fluid filled cyst is very rarely
cancerous and if it is a normal follicular cyst, it
will go away within your next three cycles. A
complex cyst is also most likely benign but cancer
usually comes in the form of a complex cyst so it is
usually recommended that these be removed and
biopsied, just to be on the safe side.

Unfortunately, the symptoms of ovarian cancer are
extremely vague and could also be other things
such as bowel issues and PMS. This is why it is so

difficult to diagnose based on symptoms. There is a blood test called the CA-125 which tests for a specific cancer antigen that is present in large numbers when ovarian cancer is present (anything under 35 is considered normal and usually ovarian cancer cases present in the hundreds). However, this test is notoriously unreliable in pre-menopausal women and can show cancer when none is present or miss stage 1 ovarian cancer. The test is much more accurate in post-menopausal women.

If your cyst is around 5 cm and it is only filled with fluid, then it is highly unlikely that you have cancer. Usually a gynecologist would recommend that you have a follow-up ultrasound in three menstrual cycles to ensure that the cyst is gone. If the cyst is a complex cyst, all will depend upon the radiologist's report. Some complex cysts can be identified as "chocolate" cysts (filled with blood) or "dermoid" cysts (filled with hair and teeth) and others may even look sinister to the well trained eye.

Pathological cysts

The incidence of ovarian carcinoma (malignant cancer) is approximately 15 cases per 100,000 women per year.[8]

Other cysts are pathological, such as those found in polycystic ovary syndrome, or those associated with tumors.

A polycystic-appearing ovary is diagnosed based on its enlarged size—usually twice normal—with small cysts present around the outside of the ovary. It can be found in "normal" women, and in women with endocrine disorders. An ultrasound is used to view the ovary in diagnosing the condition. Polycystic-appearing ovary is different from the polycystic ovarian syndrome, which includes other symptoms in addition to the presence of ovarian cysts, and involves metabolic and cardiovascular risks linked to insulin resistance. These risks include increased glucose intolerance, Type 2 diabetes, and high blood pressure. Polycystic ovarian syndrome is associated with infertility, abnormal bleeding, increased incidences of pregnancy loss, and pregnancy-related complications. Polycystic ovarian syndrome is extremely common, is thought to occur in 4–7% of women of reproductive age, and is associated with an increased risk for endometrial cancer. More tests than an ultrasound alone are required to diagnose polycystic ovarian syndrome.

I have severe pain in my right side and in my lower back. I have gained a few pounds and I

am always tired. The doctor found a cyst on my ovary that was an inch big about one year ago. Could this be ovarian cancer?

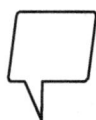

Most ovarian cysts are benign and will resolve by themselves, and they can cause the symptoms that you mention. However, you need to have a follow-up with your doctor just to be sure everything is okay.

I had cysts on my ovaries for several years. Last year, I was having all of the symptoms of ovarian cancer - fatigue, bloating, weight loss, pain, etc. An ultrasound showed that one of my cysts had become a solid mass. I had surgery to remove my ovaries and everything was benign. My symptoms have all disappeared since then.

Symptoms

Some or all of the following symptoms may be present, though it is possible not to experience any symptoms:

• Dull aching, or severe, sudden, and sharp pain or discomfort in the lower abdomen (one or both sides), pelvis, vagina, lower back, or thighs; pain may be constant or intermittent -- this is the most common symptom

- Fullness, heaviness, pressure, swelling, or bloating in the abdomen

- Breast tenderness

- Pain during or shortly after beginning or end of menstrual period.

- Irregular periods, or abnormal uterine bleeding or spotting

- Change in frequency or ease of urination (such as inability to fully empty the bladder), or difficulty with bowel movements due to pressure on adjacent pelvic anatomy

- Weight gain

- Nausea or vomiting

- Fatigue

- Infertility

- Increased level of hair growth

- Increased facial hair or body hair

- Headaches

- Strange pains in ribs, which feel muscular

- Bloating

- Strange nodules that feel like bruises under the layer of skin[9][10][11][12][13]

I was just wondering if anyone out there has the same pain that I do. I have ovarian cysts, and I've been having this pain for more than two years now. I have bad pelvic pain low back pain that goes down my thighs. Also, I'm always bloated, experience pain when I have a bowel, heavy periods. My doctor thinks this pain is not caused by my cysts.

I had the exact same symptoms as you for three years. It's from the cysts. Find a new doctor who will perform surgery on you to have them removed.

Treatment

About 95% of ovarian cysts are benign, meaning they are not cancerous.[14]

Treatment for cysts depends on the size of the cyst and symptoms. For small, asymptomatic cysts, the wait and see approach with regular check-ups will most likely be recommended.

Pain caused by ovarian cysts may be treated with:

- pain relievers, including acetaminophen (Tylenol), nonsteroidal anti-inflammatory drugs such as ibuprofen (Motrin, Advil), or narcotic pain medicine (by prescription) may help reduce pelvic pain.[15] NSAIDs usually work best when taken at the first signs of the pain.

- a warm bath, heating pad, or hot water bottle applied to the lower abdomen near the ovaries can relax tense muscles and relieve cramping, lessen discomfort, and stimulate circulation and healing in the ovaries.[16] Bags of ice covered with towels can be used alternately as cold treatments to increase local circulation.[17]

- chamomile herbal tea (Matricaria recutita) can reduce ovarian cyst pain and soothe tense muscles.[18][19]

- urinating as soon as the urge presents itself.[18]

- avoiding constipation, which does not cause ovarian cysts but may further increase pelvic discomfort.[18]

- in diet, eliminating caffeine and alcohol, reducing sugars, increasing foods rich in vitamin A and carotenoids (e.g., carrots, tomatoes, and salad greens) and B vitamins (e.g., whole grains).[17]

- combined methods of hormonal contraception such as the combined oral contraceptive pill -- the hormones in the pills may regulate the menstrual cycle, prevent the formation of follicles that can turn into cysts, and possibly shrink an existing cyst. (American College of Obstetricians and Gynecologists, 1999c; Mayo Clinic, 2002e)[15]

Also, limiting strenuous activity may reduce the risk of cyst rupture or torsion.

Cysts that persist beyond two or three menstrual cycles, or occur in post-menopausal women, may indicate more serious disease and should be investigated through ultrasonography and laparoscopy, especially in cases where family members have had ovarian cancer. Such cysts may require surgical biopsy. Additionally, a blood test may be taken before surgery to check for elevated CA-125, a tumor marker, which is often found in increased levels in ovarian cancer, although it can also be elevated by other conditions resulting in a large number of false positives.[20]

For more serious cases where cysts are large and persisting, doctors may suggest surgery. Some surgeries can be performed to successfully remove the cyst(s) without hurting the ovaries, while others may require removal of one or both ovaries.

My wife was recently diagnosed with an ovarian cyst at 5.5 cm, the size the surgeon recommends removal. However, she also has a large fibroid near the top of her uterus (that is actually interfering with the ultrasound results for the cyst).

She has suffered from irregular and very heavy periods for several years now, including severe to debilitating pain and heavy bleeding and discharge. She is now 44 and a visit last year to an endocrinologist diagnosed her as peri-menopausal.

We are currently waiting for the results of blood tests and a endometrial biopsy. The surgeon is recommending a laparoscopic procedure to remove the cyst, and likely remove the entire ovary, and to do a frozen section on the second ovary to check for irregularities. However, due to the fibroid, whose position and size is not conducive to removal techniques, the surgeon is also recommending a super cervical hysterectomy (also done as a lap procedure).

His recommendation for this was to address my wife's difficult periods.

I was just wondering if anyone has been in a situation close to this and would like to share their story or advice.

I don't have a lot of information on your wife's situation. I've had some cysts, but most of them have resolved (even one composite cyst) and I don't know their sizes. I recently had a LAVH (laparoscopically assisted vaginal hysterectomy) as treatment for cervical cancer (Ia1). I am really pleased with the hysterectomy.

I also had a fibroid. Back in December I had UFE (uterine fibroid embolization) which was supposed to shrink my 9.3cm fibroid. I think my gynecologist/oncologist said the fibroid was at 8cm when she did the hysterectomy, so it didn't shrink very much. This means when my doctor did my surgery, she had to pull out my 8cm uterus plus its 8cm fibroid. She said she had a difficult time getting the uterus out.

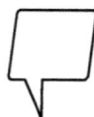

Over the years I have had fibroids and some have been painful. None were as large as your wife's. My first doctor recommended I have a

hysterectomy. After a little research, I found out that fibroids often shrink after menopause. I went to another doctor and he said he would surgically take out the fibroids. I said I would wait as I was starting to go through menopause. Well, for me, that was a good decision. One fibroid is completely gone and the other two have shrunk to the point where I no longer have any pain.

GERM CELL TUMOR

A germ cell tumor (GCT) is a neoplasm derived from germ cells. Germ cell tumors can be cancerous or non-cancerous tumors. Germ cells normally occur inside the gonads (ovary and testis). Germ cell tumors that originate outside the gonads may be birth defects resulting from errors during development of the embryo.

Etiology

Some investigators suggest that this distribution arises as a consequence of abnormal migration of germ cells during embryogenesis. Others hypothesize a widespread distribution of germ cells to multiple sites during normal embryogenesis, with these cells conveying genetic information or providing regulatory functions at somatic sites.

Extragonadal germ cell tumors were thought initially to be isolated metastases from an undetected primary tumor in a gonad, but it is now known that many germ cell tumors are congenital and originate outside the gonads. The most notable of these is sacrococcygeal teratoma, the single most common tumor diagnosed in babies at birth.

Classification

Germ cell tumors are classified by their histology,[1] regardless of location in the body.

Germ cell tumors are broadly divided in two classes:[2]

- The germinomatous or seminomatous germ cell tumors (GGCT, SGCT) include only germinoma and its synonyms dysgerminoma and seminoma.

- The nongerminomatous or nonseminomatous germ cell tumors (NGGCT, NSGCT) include all other germ cell tumors, pure and mixed.

The two classes reflect an important clinical difference. Compared to germinomatous tumors, nongerminomatous tumors tend to grow faster, have an earlier mean age at time of diagnosis (~25 years versus ~35 years, in the case of testicular cancers), and have a lower five-year survival rate. The survival rate for germinomatous tumors is higher in part because these tumors are exquisitely sensitive to radiation, and they also respond well to chemotherapy. The prognosis for nongerminomatous has improved dramatically, however, due to the use of platinum-based chemotherapy regimens.[3]

Teratocarcinoma refers to a germ cell tumor that is a mixture of teratoma with embryonal carcinoma, or with choriocarcinoma, or with both.[4] This kind of mixed germ cell tumor may be known simply as a teratoma with elements of embryonal carcinoma or choriocarcinoma, or simply by ignoring the teratoma component and referring only to its malignant component: embryonal carcinoma and/or choriocarcinoma.

Location

Despite their name, germ cell tumors occur both within and outside the ovary and testis.

- head

- inside the cranium — pineal and suprasellar locations are most commonly reported

- inside the mouth — a fairly common location for teratoma

- neck

- 1% to 5% in the mediastinum (mediastinal germ cell tumor)

- pelvis, particularly sacrococcygeal teratoma

- ovary

- testis

In females, germ cell tumors account for 30% of ovarian tumors, but only 1 to 3% of ovarian cancers in North America. In younger women germ cell tumors are more common, thus in patients under the age of 21, 60% of ovarian tumors are of the germ cell type, and up to one-third are malignant. In males, germ cell tumors of the testis occur typically after puberty and are malignant (testicular cancer). In neonates, infants, and children younger than four years, the majority of germ cell tumors are sacrococcygeal teratomas.

Males with Klinefelter's syndrome have a 50 times greater risk of germ cell tumors (GSTs).[5] In these persons, germ cell tumors usually contain nonseminomatous elements, present at an earlier age, and seldom are gonadal in location.

Prognosis

The 1997 International Germ Cell Consensus Classification[6] is a tool for estimating the risk of relapse after treatment of malignant germ cell tumor.

A small study of ovarian tumors in girls[7] reports a correlation between cystic and benign tumors and, conversely, solid and malignant tumors. Because the cystic extent of a tumor can be estimated by ultrasound, MRI, or CT scan before surgery, this permits selection of the most appropriate surgical plan to minimize risk of spillage of a malignant tumor.

Research

Germ cell tumors of children are the subject of clinical research by the worldwide Children's Oncology Group (COG), in a number of studies coordinated by Dr. John Cullen, MD.[8]

Intracranial Germ Cell Tumors have been studied through the International CNS GCT Study Group. Under the direction of Jonathan Finlay, the program director, three international treatment studies have been initiated since 1990 with the goal to maintain a high rate of cure while minimizing the late effects of treatment.

DESMOPLASTIC SMALL ROUND CELL TUMOR

Desmoplastic small round cell tumor is classified as a soft tissue sarcoma. It is an aggressive and rare tumor that primarily occurs as masses in the abdomen.[1] Other areas affected may include the lymph nodes, the lining of the abdomen, diaphragm, spleen, liver, chest wall, skull, spinal cord, large intestine, small intestine, bladder, brain, lungs, testicles, ovaries, and the pelvis. Reported sites of metatastic spread include the liver, lungs, lymph nodes, brain, skull, and bones.

The tumor is considered a childhood cancer that predominantly strikes boys and young adults.

The disease rarely occurs in females, but when it does the tumors can be mistaken for ovarian cancer.[2]

Causes

There are no known risk factors that have been identified specific to the disease. The tumor appears to arise from the primitive cells of childhood, and is considered a childhood cancer.

Research has indicated that there is a chimerical relationship between desmoplastic small round cell tumor and Wilm's tumor and Ewing's sarcoma.

Desmoplastic small round cell tumor is associated with a unique chromosomal translocation (t11;22)(p13:q12)[3] resulting in a EWS/WT1 transcript[4] that is diagnostic of this tumor.[1] This transcript codes for a protein that acts as a transcriptional activator that fails to suppress tumor growth.

The EWS/WT1 translocation product targets ENT4.[5] ENT4 is also known as PMAT.

There is an association between desmoid tumors and Gardner's syndrome, a variant of Familial adenomatous polyposis with extra-colonic manifestations.[6]

Symptoms

There are few early warning signs that a patient has a desmoplastic small round cell tumor. Patients are often young and healthy as the tumors grow and spread uninhibited within the abdominal cavity. These are rare tumors and symptoms are often misdiagnosed by family physicians. The abdominal masses can grow to enormous size before being noticed by the patient. The tumors can be felt as hard, round masses by palpating the abdomen.

First symptoms of the disease often include abdominal distention, abdominal mass, abdominal or back pain, gastrointestinal obstruction, lack of appetite, ascites, anemia, and/or cachexia.

Other reported symptoms include unknown lumps, thyroid conditions, hormonal conditions, blood clotting, kidney or urological problems, testicle, breast, uterine, vaginal, or ovarian masses.

Differentials

Because this is a rare tumor not many family physicians or oncologists are familiar with this disease. Desmoplastic small round cell tumor in young patients can be mistaken for other abdominal tumors including rhabdomyosarcoma, neuroblastoma, and mesenteric carcinoid. In older patients desmoplastic small round cell tumor can resemble lymphoma, peritoneal mesothelioma, and peritoneal carcinomatosis. In males desmoplastic small round cell tumor may be mistaken for germ cell or testicular cancer. In females desmoplastic small round cell tumor can be mistaken for Ovarian cancer. Desmoplastic small round cell tumor shares characteristics with other small round cell cancers including Ewing's sarcoma, acute leukemia, small cell mesothelioma, neuroblastoma, primitive neuroectodermal tumor, rhabdomyosarcoma, and Wilm's tumor.

Pathology

Pathology reveals well circumscribed solid tumor nodules within a dense desmoplastic stroma. Often areas of central necrosis are present. Tumor cells have hyperchromatic nuclei with increased nuclear/cytoplasmic ratio.

On immunohistochemistry, these cells have trilinear coexpression including the epithelial marker cytokeratin, the mesenchymal markers desmin and vimentin, and the neuronal marker neuron-specific enolase. Thus, although initially thought to be of mesothelial origin due to sites of presentation, it is now hypothesized to arise from a progenitor cell with multiphenotypic differentiation.

Treatment

Desmoplastic small round cell tumor is frequently misdiagnosed. Adult patients should always be referred to a sarcoma specialist. This is an aggressive, rare, fast spreading tumor and both pediatric and adult patients should be treated at a sarcoma center.

There is no standard protocol for the disease.[7] However, recent journals and studies have reported that some patients respond to high dose (P6 Protocol) chemotherapy, maintenance chemotherapy, debulking operation, cytoreductive surgery, and radiation therapy. Other treatment options include: hematopoietic stem cell transplantation, intensity-modulated radiation Therapy, radiofrequency ablation, stereotactic body radiation therapy, intraperitoneal hyperthermic chemoperfusion, and clinical trials.

Prognosis

The prognosis for desmoplastic small round cell tumor remains poor[8] with less than 20% surviving beyond two to three years.[citation needed] Prognosis often depends upon the stage of the cancer and the grade of the tumor. Because the disease can be misdiagnosed or remain undetected tumors frequently grow large within the abdomen and metastasized or seed to other parts of the body.

There is no known organ or area of origin. Desmoplastic small round cell tumor can metastasize through lymph nodes or the blood stream. Sites of metastatis include the spleen, diaphragm, liver, large and small intestine, lungs, central nervous system, bones, uterus, bladder, genitals, abdominal cavity, and the brain.

A multi-modality approach of high dose chemotherapy, aggressive surgical resection,[7] radiation, and stem cell rescue improves survival for some patients. Reports have indicated that patients will initially respond to first line chemotherapy and treatment but that relapse is common.

Some patients in remission or with inoperable tumor seem to benefit from long term low dose chemotherapy, turning desmoplastic small round cell tumor into a chronic disease.

Research

The Stehlin Foundation[9] currently offers desmoplastic small round cell tumor patients the opportunity to send samples of their tumors free of charge for testing. Research scientists are growing the samples on nude mice and testing various chemical agents to find which are most effective against the individual's tumor.

Patients with advanced desmoplastic small round cell tumor may qualify to participate in clinical trials that are researching new drugs to treat the disease.

SURFACE EPITHELIAL – STROMAL TUMORS

Surface epithelial-stromal tumors are a class of ovarian neoplasms that may be benign or malignant. Neoplasms in this group are thought to be derived from the ovarian surface epithelium (modified peritoneum) or from ectopic endometrial or Fallopian tube (tubal) tissue. This group of tumors accounts for the majority of all ovarian tumors. Serum CA-125 is often elevated but is only 50% accurate so it is not a useful tumor marker to assess the progress of treatment.

Classification

Epithelial-stromal tumors are classified on the basis of the epithelial cell type, the relative amounts of epithelium and stroma, the presence of papillary processes, and the location of the epithelial elements. Microscopic pathological features determine whether a surface epithelial-stromal tumor is benign, borderline, or malignant (evidence of malignancy and stromal invasion). Borderline tumors are of uncertain malignant potential.

This group consists of serous, mucinous, endometrioid, clear cell, and brenner (transitional cell) tumors, though there are a few mixed, undifferentiated and unclassified types.

Serous tumors

- These tumors vary in size from small and nearly imperceptible to large, filling the abdominal cavity.

- Benign, borderline, and malignant types of serous tumors account for about 30% of all ovarian tumors.

- 75% are benign or of borderline malignancy, and 25% are malignant

- The malignant form of this tumor, serous cystadenocarcinoma, accounts for approximately 40% of all carcinomas of the ovary and are the most common malignant ovarian tumors.

- Benign and borderline tumors are most common between the ages of 20 and 50 years.

- Malignant serous tumors occur later in life on average, although somewhat earlier in familial cases.

- 20% of benign, 30% of borderline, and 66% of malignant tumors are bilateral (affect both ovaries).

Components can include:

1. cystic areas

2. cystic and fibrous areas

3. predominantly fibrous areas

The chance of malignancy of the tumor increases with the amount of solid areas present, including both papillary structures and any necrotic tissue present.

Pathology

• lined by tall, columnar, ciliated epithelial cells

• filled with clear serous fluid

• the term serous which originated as a description of the cyst fluid has come to be describe the particular type of epithelial cell seen in these tumors

• may involve the surface of the ovary

• the division between benign, borderline, and malignant is ascertained by assessing:

• cellular atypia (whether or not individual cells look abnormal)

• invasion of surrounding ovarian stroma (whether or not cells are infiltrating surrounding tissue)

• borderline tumors may have cellular atypia but do NOT have evidence of invasion

- the presence of psammoma bodies are a characteristic microscopic finding of cystadenocarcinomas[1]

Prognosis

The prognosis of a serous tumor, like most neoplasms, depends on

- degree of differentiation

  - this is how closely the tumor cells resemble benign cells

  - a well-differentiated tumor closely resembles benign tumors

  - a poorly differentiated tumor may not resemble the cell type of origin at all

  - a moderately differentiated tumor usually resembles the cell type of origin, but appears frankly malignant

- extension of tumor to other structures

  - in particular with serous malignancies, the presence of malignant spread to the peritoneum is important with regard to prognosis.

The five year survival rate of borderline and malignant tumors confined to the ovaries are 100%

and 70% respectively. If the peritoneum is involved, these rates become 90% and 25%.

While the 5-year survival rates of borderline tumors are excellent, this should not be seen as evidence of cure, as recurrences can occur many years later.

Mucinous tumors

Mucinous tumors:

- Closely resemble their serous counterparts

- Somewhat less common, accounting for about 25% of all ovarian neoplasms

- Occur principally in middle adult life and are rare before puberty and after menopause

- 80% are benign or borderline and about 15% are malignant

- Mucinous cystadenocarcinomas (the malignant form of this tumor) are relatively uncommon and account for only 10% of all ovarian cancers

- Mucinous tumors are characterized by more cysts of variable size and a rarity of surface involvement as compared to serous tumors

- Also in comparison to serous tumors, mucinous tumors are less frequently bilateral, approximately 5% of primary mucinous tumors are bilateral.

- May form very large cystic masses, with recorded weights exceeding 25kg

- Appear as multiloculated tumors filled with sticky, gelatinous fluid

Pathology

Benign mucinous tumors are characterized by a lining of tall columnar epithelial cells with apical mucin and the absence of cilia, similar in appearance with benign cervical or intestinal epithelia. Cystadenocarcinomas (malignant tumors) contain a more solid growth pattern with the hallmarks of malignancy: cellular atypia and stratification, loss of the normal architecture of the tissue, and necrosis. The appearance can look similar to colonic cancer. Clear stromal invasion is used to differentiate borderline tumors from malignant tumors.

Prognosis

10-year survival rates for borderline tumors contained within the ovary, malignant tumors without invasion, and invasive malignant tumors are greater than 95%, 90%, and 66%, respectively.

One rare but noteworthy condition associated with mucinous ovarian neoplasms is pseudomyxoma peritonei. As primary ovarian mucinous tumors are usually unilateral (in one ovary), the presentation of bilateral mucinous tumors requires exclusion of a non-ovarian origin.

Endometrioid tumors

Endometrioid tumors account for approximately 20% of all ovarian cancers and are mostly malignant (endometroid carcinomas). They are made of tubular glands bearing a close resemblance to benign or malignant endometrium. 15–30% of endometrioid carcinomas occur in individuals with carcinoma of the endometrium, and these patients have a better prognosis. They appear similar to other surface epithelial-stromal tumors, with solid and cystic areas. 40% of these tumors are bilateral, when bilateral, metastases is often present.

Pathology

- Glands bearing a strong resemblance to endometrial-type glands

  - Benign tumors have mature-appearing glands in a fibrous stroma

- Borderline tumors have a complex branching pattern without stromal invasion

- Carcinomas (malignant tumors) have invasive glands with crowded, atypical cells, frequent mitoses. With poorer differentiation, the tumor becomes more solid.

Prognosis

Prognosis again is dependent on the spread of the tumor, as well as how differentiated the tumor appears. The overall prognosis is somewhat worse than for serous or mucinous tumors, and the 5-year survival rate for patients with tumors confined to the ovary is approximately 75%.

Clear cell tumors

Clear cell tumors are characterized by large epithelial cells with abundant clear cytoplasm and may be seen in association with endometriosis or endometrioid carcinoma of the ovary, bearing a resemblance to clear cell carcinoma of the endometrium. They may be predominantly solid or cystic. If solid, the clear cells tend to be arranged in sheets or tubules. In the cystic variety, the neoplastic cells make up the cyst lining.

Prognosis

These tumors tend to be aggressive, the five year survival rate for tumors confined to the ovaries is approximately 65%. If the tumor has spread beyond the ovary at diagnosis, the prognosis is poor

Brenner tumor

Brenner tumors are uncommon surface-epithelial stromal cell tumors in which the epithelial cell (which defines these tumors) is a transitional cell. These are similar in appearance to bladder epithelia. The tumors may be very small to very large, and may be solid or cystic. Histologically, the tumor consists of nests of the aforementioned transitional cells within surrounding tissue that resembles normal ovary. Brenner tumors may be benign or malignant, depending on whether the tumor cells invade the surrounding tissue.

Treatment

For advanced cancer of this histology, the US National Cancer Institute recommends a method of chemotherapy that combines intravenous (IV) and intraperitoneal (IP) administration.[2] Preferred chemotherapeutic agents include a platinum drug with a taxane.

SEX CORD – GONADAL STROMAL TUMOR

Sex cord-gonadal stromal tumor (or sex cord-stromal tumor) is a group of tumors of sex cord-derived tissues of the ovary and testis. In humans, this group accounts for 8% of ovarian cancers and under 5% of testicular cancers. Their diagnosis is histological: only a biopsy of the tumour can make an exact diagnosis. They are often suspected of being malignant prior to operation, being solid ovarian tumors that tend to occur most commonly in post menopausal women.

This group of tumors is significantly less common than testicular germ cell tumors in men,[1] and slightly less common than ovarian germ cell tumors in women.

Tumor types in order of prevalence

• Granulosa cell tumor. This tumor produces granulosa cells, which normally are found in the ovary. It is malignant in 20% of women diagnosed with it. It tends to present in women in the 50–55yo age group with post menopausal vaginal bleeding. Uncommonly, a similar but possibly distinct tumor, juvenile granulosa cell tumor, presents in pre-pubertal girls with precocious puberty. In both groups, the vaginal bleeding is due to oestrogen secreted by the tumor. In older women, treatment is total abdominal hysterectomy and removal of both ovaries. In young girls, fertility sparing treatment is the mainstay for non-metastatic disease.

- Sertoli cell tumor. This tumor produces Sertoli cells, which normally are found in the testicle. This tumor occurs in both men and women.

- Thecoma. This tumor produces theca of follicle, a tissue normally found in the ovarian follicle. The tumor is almost exclusively benign and unilateral. It typically secretes androgens, and as a result women with this tumor often present with new onset of hirsutism or virilisation.

- Leydig cell tumor. This tumor produces Leydig cells, which normally are found in the testicle and tend to secrete androgens.

- Sertoli-Leydig cell tumor. This tumor produces both Sertoli and Leydig cells. Although both cell types normally occur in the testicle, this tumour can occur in the ovary.

- Gynandroblastoma. A very rare tumor producing both ovarian (granulosa and/or theca) and testicular (Sertoli and/or Leydig) cells or tissues. Typically it consists of adult-type granulosa cells and Sertoli cells,[2][3] but it has been reported with juvenile-type granulosa cells.[4] It has been reported to occur in the ovary usually, rarely in the testis.[5] Due to its rarity, the malignant potential of this tumor is unclear; there is one case report of late metastasis.

Diagnosis

Definitive diagnosis of these tumors is based on the histology of tissue obtained in a biopsy or surgical resection. In a retrospective study of 72 cases in children and adolescents, the histology was important to prognosis.[6]

A number of molecules have been proposed as markers for this group of tumors. CD56 may be useful for distinguishing sex cord-stromal tumors from some other types of tumors, although it does not distinguish them from neuroendocrine tumors.[7] Calretinin has also been suggested as a marker.[8] For diagnosis of granulosa cell tumor, inhibin is under investigation.

On magnetic resonance imaging, a fibroma may produce one of several imaging features that might be used in the future to identify this rare tumor prior to surgery.[9][10]

Prognosis

A retrospective study of 83 women with sex cord-stromal tumours (73 with granulosa cell tumour and 10 with Sertoli-Leydig cell tumor), all diagnosed between 1975 and 2003, reported that survival was higher with age under 50, smaller tumour size, and absence of residual disease. The study found no effect of chemotherapy.[11] A retrospective study of 67 children and adolescents reported some benefit of cisplatin-based chemotherapy.[12]

Research

A prospective study of ovarian sex cord-stromal tumors in children and adolescents began enrolling participants in 2005.[12]

FOLLICULAR CYST OF OVARY

One type of simple cyst, which is the most common type of ovarian cyst, is the follicular cyst of ovary, or *graafian follicle cyst*, or *follicular cyst*. This type can form when ovulation doesn't occur, and a follicle doesn't rupture or release its egg but instead grows until it becomes a cyst, or when a mature follicle involutes (collapses on itself). It usually forms during ovulation, and can grow to about 6cm (2.3 inches) in diameter. It is thin-walled, lined by one or more layers of granulosa cell, and filled with clear fluid. Its rupture can create sharp, severe pain on the side of the ovary on which the cyst appears. This sharp pain (sometimes called mittelschmerz) occurs in the middle of the menstrual cycle, during ovulation. About a fourth of women with this type of cyst experience pain. Usually, these cysts produce no symptoms and disappear by themselves within a few months. Ultrasound is the primary tool used to document the follicular cyst. A pelvic exam will also aid in the diagnosis if the cyst is large enough to be seen. A doctor monitors these to make sure they disappear, and looks at treatment options if they do not.

Could someone give me some more information on ovarian cysts? I was just told I have a

"resolving ovarian cyst". I am unsure what that means. Will this happen every month? I have had this pain off and on for years; does that mean that I keep getting cysts? I had such bad pain in my lower right front and back and it felt like I was bleeding inside- it felt so hot; does that mean rupture? Can a cyst cause diarrhea? Does having cysts put you at more of a risk for cancer?

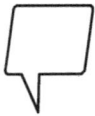

I know you must be relieved to find that you don't have cancer, though cysts can still cause a lot of problems, even though they are not as serious. Ovarian cysts are very common in women of childbearing years. Every month when you ovulate, there is a small fluid-filled bubble on your ovaries that contains the egg. When the egg is released, usually that bubble will collapse and shrink, but occasionally they don't and they continue to grow. These lingering fluid-filled cysts are called functional cysts. They can become very large and cause a lot of different symptoms, such as pain in the abdomen and even up into the shoulder, bloating, constipation, diarrhea, abnormal periods, nausea, etc. In most cases, these cysts will resolve within a few months on their own. If they don't, then there are medications which can be given or surgery can be performed to either remove just the cyst or to remove the entire ovary.

Sometimes cysts display "abnormal" characteristics such as walls within the cysts or solid components. These are called complex cysts. They can be more troublesome and in rare cases can be cancerous. They also may take longer to resolve or disappear.

Ruptured cysts can cause severe pain, fever, and vomiting. If this occurs, you should see your doctor as soon as possible.

Ovarian cysts can occur at any time, though they may not cause the same problems each time. There may be times you don't even know that you have a cyst and there may be times that a very small cyst causes a lot of pain and other symptoms. It does seem that some women are more prone to cysts. There is even a condition called polycystic ovarian syndrome in which a woman might have many cysts form each month.

I had a CT scan to help figure out why I've been having vomit/diarrhea for over two weeks. They could not find anything. Instead, they found I had womanly issues. I was told to see gynecologist ASAP. Can anyone offer any insight in what these *findings mean so I have an idea before seeing the gynecologist?*

Here is the report for CT Scan:

CT examination of the pelvis was performed. The uterus is anteverted. The uterus measures approximately 11.3 cm x 6.5 cm x 7.7 cm. There is some lobular appearance of the cervix. There is some fluid in the endometrial canal. I cannot exclude cervical pathology. Consider further evaluations and direct inspection. The adnexa areas are reviewed. There is a small left ovarian follicular cyst measuring approximately 1 cm in size. There is however asymmetrical bulbous appearance to the cervix. It has concave margins and there is suggestion of fluid within the endocervical canal. Cervical pathology cannot be excluded. There is a 1 cm left ovarian follicular cyst. Consider follow up studies and direct inspection.

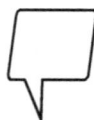

First of all, an anteverted uterus is nothing at all. Mine is retroverted. This simply means that your uterus is slightly "skewed", and many women have this.

Second of all, follicular ovarian cysts are completely normal cysts that all of us grow on our ovaries every month. They contain our eggs and these come and go with our normal cycle. The measurement of 1 cm is completely within the norm of a follicular cyst so this just means you are ovulating normally.

The area of concern is therefore your cervical canal, where the radiologist seems to see fluid buildup. All the report states is that your cervix seems to have an unusual shape and because of this, the radiologist cannot exclude the need for further tests, such as a direct inspection by a gynecologist. He does not seem to mention any lesions or tumors either in either your uterus or your cervix but I am not sure how well a CT scan can see these things.

See if you can get an ultrasound done as this will be able to see the thickness of the lining of your uterus and also what the fluid in the endocervical canal is. Perhaps you can see a gynecologist who also does internal ultrasounds. This would be ideal as you can have the results while the gynecologist is performing the test. You will most likely also need to have a pap smear, an endometrial biopsy and perhaps an HPV test.

The report you have is very inconclusive so don't let this worry you. Sometimes these radiologists don't see a textbook image (which none of us are, by the way) and they therefore cannot exclude anything. An ultrasound will offer a much better image of what is actually there.

BRENNER TUMOR

Brenner tumors are uncommon tumors that are part of the surface epithelial-stromal tumor group of ovarian neoplasms.

The majority of these tumors are benign. However, they can be malignant.[1]

They are most frequently found as incidental findings[2] on pelvic examination or at laparotomy.

Brenner tumors very rarely can occur in other locations, including testis

Presentation

On gross pathological examination, they are solid, sharply circumscribed and pale yellow-tan in color. 90% are unilateral (arising in one ovary, the other is unaffected). The tumors can vary in size from less than 1 cm to 30 cm. Borderline and malignant Brenner tumors are possible but each are rare.

Diagnosis

Histologically, there are nests of transitional-type epithelial cells with longitudinal nuclear grooves (coffee bean nuclei) lying in abundant fibrous stroma.

KRUKENBERG TUMOR

A Krukenberg tumor classically refers to a metastatic ovarian malignancy whose primary site arose in the gastrointestinal tract or breast. Diffuse gastric carcinoma (linitis plastica) used to be the most common, but lately there have been an increase in breast origin.[1] Krukenberg tumors are often found in both ovaries. Microscopically, they are characterized by appearance of mucin-secreting signet-ring cells in the tissue of the ovary; when the primary tumor is discovered, the same signet-ring cells are typically found.

Historical

The Krukenberg tumor is named after Friedrich Ernst Krukenberg (1871-1946),[2] a German doctor who first described them as "fibrosarcoma ovarii mucocellulare carcinomatodes".[3]

Etiology and Incidence

Metastatic cancer of the ovary accounts for only about 5% of ovarian cancer; in the remainder, the ovary is the primary cancer site. Krukenberg tumors are the third most common metastatic ovarian cancer (after epithelial and germ-cell tumors) and make up 14% of these cancers. Unlike some forms of cancer, there is no racial bias. Krukenberg tumors are most commonly seen in middle-aged and elderly females, around or following menopause.

Symptoms

Patients with Krukenberg tumor often come to the attention of their doctor when they present complaining of abdominal or pelvic pain, bloatedness, vaginal bleeding, a change in their menstrual habit or pain during intercourse. These symptoms are non-specific (i.e., they point to a range of problems other than cancer) and a diagnosis can only be made following Computed Tomography (CT) scans, laparotomy and/or a biopsy of the ovary.

Pathogenesis

There is some debate over the exact mechanism of metastasis of the tumor cells from the stomach, appendix or colon to the ovaries; classically it was thought that direct seeding across the abdominal cavity accounted for the spread of this tumor, but recently some researchers have suggested that lymphatic (i.e. through the lymph nodes), or haematogenous (i.e. through the blood) spread is more likely, as most of these tumors are found on the inside of the ovaries. Proponents of this theory cite the fact that metastases are never found in the omentum (the fatty apron which envelops the organs of the abdomen and lies between the stomach and ovaries), and that the tumor cells are found within the ovary and not growing inwards. However, this remains a controversy, as cases in Hong Kong always showed omental spread and peritoneal seedlings in patients with Krukenberg tumors.

Although a Krukenberg tumor is most commonly a metastasis from a gastric cancer (usually an adenocarcinoma), this is not always the case. Other tumors of the gastrointestinal tract (including, significantly, colon cancer) have been known to cause Krukenberg tumors, and recent case-reports of Krukenberg tumors originating from tumors of the tip of the appendix have appeared in the medical literature. A metastatic tumor originating in the breast may also fit the category of Krukenberg tumor if it expresses intracellular mucin and displays positive immunohistochemical staining with epithelial markers.[4]

Treatment and Prognosis

Since the Krukenberg tumor is a secondary (metastatic) tumor, management of the tumor must involve finding and treating the primary cancer. In general, most cases of Krukenberg tumor have a poor prognosis and radical operation such as removal of the ovaries (and the colon or appendix if involved) can improve survival only in cases of solitary ovarian metastasis or local extended disease (i.e. the lesion is located only in the pelvis). Cancer chemotherapy and radiotherapy before surgery may be used to shrink the tumor and facilitate its removal.

PRIMARY PERITONEAL CANCER

Primary peritoneal cancer or carcinoma ("PPCa")[1] is a cancer of the cells lining the peritoneum, or abdominal cavity.

Some studies indicate that 7–20% of initially diagnosed epithelial ovarian cancers could be properly reclassified as primary peritoneal cancers.

I had my follow-up Transvaginal Ultrasound. From what the technician was able to tell me, it is now a 3.8 cm simple cyst (was a little under 3 cm). The walls seem a little thicker, so it might have a small "complex". Are thicker walls a bad thing? She told me it did not have any characteristics of being a cancer cyst. Normally, she said when they see a cancerous cyst there is no doubting it, and to her this looks completely benign, but this is just her opinion as she is not a doctor.

My endometrial walls have slightly darker coloring in some spots, which could be the polyps that they diagnosed me with, but she was unable to say.

Now, ovarian cancer is going through my mind like crazy. Does this sound like I should be worried? I did gain a few pounds in the past two months (about four), but I blamed this on my junk I'm eating, and the birth control she put me on. If something was wrong would something show up in one of those tests or say my blood work?

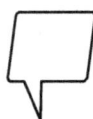

I had the same thing happen with my ovarian cyst when I was watching it for that year and a half. My radiologist said that unfortunately, these cysts have a tendency to develop thicker walls as they age. In my case, I had a thickening of a few millimeters in one section of the wall of the cyst and like you, I was very worried. I was strongly reassured, however, that the cyst is still considered a "simple" cyst and that it was not dangerous.

The predictive value of a radiologist's or gynecologist's "impressions" of an ovarian cyst on ultrasound is extremely high (something around the 90% range) and this is very reassuring. This means that ovarian cancer does indeed look different most of the time. In order to give me more reassurance, my doctors recommended that I take the CA-125 blood test. The CA-125 is not as reliable as the ultrasound but I figured that if I had the two together, I could be perhaps up to 95% assured that the thing did not pose a threat.

Four pounds is not much to be concerned about, especially if you can easily explain it, as you just did. A colleague of mine had peritoneal cancer (which is virtually the same as ovarian cancer) and she gained over 35 lbs in a very short amount of time (about a month). She was unable to keep anything down so she drank "Boost" type drinks to stay alive and she had a host of bowel issues. She felt tired and drained all of the time and knew that she was very sick. They drained I don't know how many liters of fluid from her abdomen when she finally sought help.

Try to relax and not jump to any conclusions. Get a copy of the report and if you are not reassured by this and by your doctor's advice, you can request more testing to rule things out (CA-125 for more reassurance about the cyst and perhaps an endometrial biopsy regarding the uterus). There is also the option of getting a second opinion.

Causes

Although the precise causes are not known, a link with certain variants of BRCA has been described.[2]

An association with vascular endothelial growth factor has been observed.[3]

Prognosis and treatment

Prognosis and treatment is the same as for the most common variation of ovarian cancer, which is epithelial ovarian cancer.[4][5]

Elevated albumin levels have been associated with a more favorable prognosis.[6]

Mesothelioma

The cancer does involve mesothelial cells and can be medically described as mesothelioma.

REFERENCES – OVARIAN CANCER

1. EBSCO database verified by URAC; accessed from Mount Sinai Hospital, New York

2. Robert C. Young (2005). "Ch. 83, Gynecologic Malignancies". in Jameson JN, Kasper DL, Harrison TR, Braunwald E, Fauci AS, Hauser SL, Longo DL. *Harrison's principles of internal medicine* (16th ed.). New York: McGraw-Hill Medical Publishing Division. ISBN 0-07-140235-7. http://highered.mcgraw-hill.com/sites/0071402357/information_center_view0/.

3. *Gynecologic Neoplasms* at Merck Manual of Diagnosis and Therapy Professional Edition

4. Kosary, Carol L. (2007), "Chapter 16: Cancers of the Ovary", in Ries, LAG; Young, JL; Keel, GE *et al.*, *SEER Survival Monograph: Cancer Survival Among Adults: US SEER Program, 1988-2001, Patient and Tumor Characteristics,* SEER Program, **NIH Pub. No. 07-6215,** Bethesda, MD: National Cancer Institute, pp. 133–144, http://seer.cancer.gov/publications/survival/surv_ovary.pdf

5. Goff BA, Mandel L, Muntz HG, Melancon CH (November 2000). "Ovarian carcinoma diagnosis". *Cancer* **89** (10): 2068–75. doi:10.1002/1097-0142(20001115)89:10<2068::AID-CNCR6>3.0.CO;2-Z. PMID 11066047.

6. Bankhead CR, Kehoe ST, Austoker J (July 2005). "Symptoms associated with diagnosis of ovarian cancer: a systematic review". *BJOG* **112** (7): 857–65. doi:10.1111/j.1471-0528.2005.00572.x. PMID 15957984.

7. Ryerson AB, Eheman C, Burton J, *et al.* (May 2007). "Symptoms, diagnoses, and time to key diagnostic procedures among older U.S. women with ovarian cancer". *Obstet Gynecol* **109** (5): 1053–61. doi:10.1097/01.AOG.0000260392.70365.5e (inactive 2009-03-01). PMID 17470582. http://journals.lww.com/greenjournal/pages/articleviewer.aspx?year=2007&issue=05000&article=00008&type=abstract.

8. Goff BA, Mandel LS, Melancon CH, Muntz HG (June 2004). "Frequency of symptoms of ovarian cancer in women presenting to primary care clinics". *JAMA* **291** (22): 2705–12. doi:10.1001/jama.291.22.2705. PMID 15187051. http://jama.ama-assn.org/cgi/pmidlookup?view=long&pmid=15187051.

9. Chobanian N, Dietrich CS (April 2008). "Ovarian cancer". *Surg. Clin. North Am.* **88** (2): 285–99, vi. doi:10.1016/j.suc.2007.12.002. PMID 18381114. http://linkinghub.elsevier.com/retrieve/pii/S0039-6109(07)00180-6.

10. Vo C, Carney ME (December 2007). "Ovarian cancer hormonal and environmental risk effect". *Obstet. Gynecol. Clin. North Am.* **34** (4): 687–700, viii. doi:10.1016/j.ogc.2007.09.008. PMID 18061864. http://linkinghub.elsevier.com/retrieve/pii/S0889-8545(07)00090-3.

11. Bandera CA (June 2005). "Advances in the understanding of risk factors for ovarian cancer". *J Reprod Med* **50** (6): 399–406. PMID 16050564.

12. Collaborative Group on Epidemiological Studies of Ovarian Cancer, Beral V, Doll R, Hermon C, Peto R, Reeves G (January 2008). "Ovarian cancer and oral contraceptives: collaborative reanalysis of data from 45 epidemiological studies including 23,257 women with ovarian cancer and 87,303 controls". *Lancet* **371** (9609): 303–14. doi:10.1016/S0140-6736(08)60167-1. PMID 18294997.

13. Brinton, L.A., Moghissi, K.S., Scoccia, B., Westhoff, C.L., Lamb, E.J. (2005). "Ovulation induction and cancer risk". *Fertil. Steril.* **83** (2): 261–74; quiz 525–6. doi:10.1016/j.fertnstert.2004.09.016. PMID 15705362.

14. Lakhani SR, Manek S, Penault-Llorca F, *et al.* (April 2004). "Pathology of ovarian cancers in BRCA1 and BRCA2 carriers". *Clin. Cancer Res.* **10** (7): 2473–81. PMID 15073127. http://clincancerres.aacrjournals.org/cgi/pmidlookup?vie w=long&pmid=15073127.

15. BBC News Milk link to ovarian cancer risk 29 November 2004

16. Genkinger JM, Hunter DJ, Spiegelman D, *et al.* (March 2006). "Alcohol intake and ovarian cancer risk: a pooled analysis of 10 cohort studies". *British Journal of Cancer* **94** (5): 757–62. doi:10.1038/sj.bjc.6603020. PMID 16495916.

17. La Vecchia C, Negri E, Franceschi S, Parazzini F, Gentile A, Fasoli M (September 1992). "Alcohol and epithelial ovarian cancer". *Journal of Clinical Epidemiology* **45** (9): 1025–30. doi:10.1016/0895-4356(92)90119-8. PMID 1432017.

18. "Alcohol consumption and cancer risk". Bandolier. 2007-04-01. http://www. jr2.ox.ac.uk/bandolier/booth/hliving/alccan.html.

19. Bagnardi V, Blangiardo M, La Vecchia C, Corrao G (2001). "Alcohol consumption and the risk of cancer: a meta-analysis". *Alcohol Research & Health* **25** (4): 263–70. PMID 11910703. http://pubs.niaaa.nih.gov/publications/ arh25-4/263-270.htm.

20. Goff BA, Mandel LS, Drescher CW, *et al.* (2007). "Development of an ovarian cancer symptom index: possibilities for earlier detection". *Cancer* **109** (2): 221–7. doi:10.1002/cncr.22371. PMID 17154394.

21. "Ovarian Cancer Symptoms Consensus Statement" (pdf). http://www.sgo. org/publications/OvarianCancerSymptoms.pdf. Retrieved on 2007-07-19.

22. Screening for Ovarian Cancer Daniel L. Clarke-Pearson, N Engl J Med, 361:170, July 9, 2009

23. Kurman RJ, Visvanathan K, Roden R, Wu TC, Shih IeM (April 2008). "Early detection and treatment of ovarian cancer: shifting from early stage to minimal volume of disease based on a new model of carcinogenesis". *Am. J. Obstet. Gynecol.* **198** (4): 351–6. doi:10.1016/j.ajog.2008.01.005. PMID 18395030. PMC: 2532696. http://linkinghub.elsevier.com/retrieve/pii/S0002-9378(08)00020-3.

24. Partridge E, Kreimer AR, Greenlee RT, *et al.* (April 2009). "Results from four rounds of ovarian cancer screening in a randomized trial". *Obstet Gynecol* **113** (4): 775–82. doi:10.1097/AOG.0b013e31819cda77. http://meta.wkhealth.com/pt/pt-core/template-journal/lwwgateway/media/landingpage.htm?issn=0029-7844&volume=113&issue=4&spage=775.

25. Menon U, Gentry-Maharaj A, Hallett R, *et al.* (April 2009). "Sensitivity and specificity of multimodal and ultrasound screening for ovarian cancer, and stage distribution of detected cancers: results of the prevalence screen of the UK Collaborative Trial of Ovarian Cancer Screening (UKCTOCS)". *Lancet Oncol.* **10** (4): 327–40. doi:10.1016/S1470-2045(09)70026-9. PMID 19282241. http://linkinghub.elsevier.com/retrieve/pii/S1470-2045(09)70026-9.

26. Ehrlich, P.F., Teitelbaum, D.H., Hirschl, R.B., Rescorla, F. (2007). "Excision of large cystic ovarian tumors: combining minimal invasive surgery techniques and cancer surgery—the best of both worlds". *J. Pediatr. Surg.* **42** (5): 890–3. doi:10.1016/j.jpedsurg.2006.12.069. PMID 17502206.

27. McGuire WP, Markman M (December 2003). "Primary ovarian cancer chemotherapy: current standards of care". *Br. J. Cancer* **89** (Suppl 3): S3–8. doi:10.1038/sj.bjc.6601494. PMID 14661040.

28. Armstrong DK, Bundy B, Wenzel L, Huang HQ, *et al.* (January 2006). "Intraperitoneal Cisplatin and Paclitaxel in Ovarian Cancer". *NEJM* **354** (1): 34–43. doi:10.1056/NEJMoa052985. PMID 16394300. http://content.nejm.org/cgi/content/full/354/1/34.

29. Swart AM, Burdett S, Ledermann J, Mook P, Parmar MK (April 2008). "Why i.p. therapy cannot yet be considered as a standard of care for the first-line treatment of ovarian cancer: a systematic review". *Ann. Oncol.* **19** (4): 688–95. doi:10.1093/annonc/mdm518. PMID 18006894. http://annonc.oxfordjournals.org/cgi/pmidlookup?view=long&pmid=18006894.

30. Survival rates based on SEER incidence and NCHS mortality statistics, as cited by the National Cancer Institute in SEER Stat Fact Sheets - Cancer of the Ovary

31. Bast RC, Brewer M, Zou C, *et al.* (2007). "Prevention and early detection of ovarian cancer: mission impossible?". *Recent Results Cancer Res.* **174:** 91–100. PMID 17302189.

32. Catone G, Marino G, Mancuso R, Zanghì A (April 2004). "Clinicopathological features of an equine ovarian teratoma". *Reprod. Domest. Anim.* **39** (2): 65–9. doi:10.1111/j.1439-0531.2003.00476.x. PMID 15065985.

33. Lefebvre R, Theoret C, Doré M, Girard C, Laverty S, Vaillancourt D (November 2005). "Ovarian teratoma and endometritis in a mare". *Can. Vet. J.* **46** (11): 1029–33. PMID 16363331.

34. Son YS, Lee CS, Jeong WI, Hong IH, Park SJ, Kim TH, Cho EM, Park TI, Jeong KS (May 2005). "Cystadenocarcinoma in the ovary of a Thoroughbred mare". *Aust. Vet. J.* **83** (5): 283–4. doi:10.1111/j.1751-0813.2005.tb12740.x. PMID 15957389.

35. Frederico LM, Gerard MP, Pinto CR, Gradil CM (May 2007). "Bilateral occurrence of granulosa-theca cell tumors in an Arabian mare". *Can. Vet. J.* **48** (5): 502–5. PMID 17542368.

36. Hoque S, Derar RI, Osawa T, Taya K, Watanabe G, Miyake Y (June 2003). "Spontaneous repair of the atrophic contralateral ovary without ovariectomy in the case of a granulosa theca cell tumor (GTCT) affected mare" ([dead link] – Scholar search). *J. Vet. Med. Sci.* **65** (6): 749–51. doi:10.1292/jvms.65.749. PMID 12867740. http://joi.jlc.jst.go.jp/JST.JSTAGE/jvms/65.749?from=PubMed.

37. Sedrish SA, McClure JR, Pinto C, Oliver J, Burba DJ (November 1997). "Ovarian torsion associated with granulosa-theca cell tumor in a mare". *J. Am. Vet. Med. Assoc.* **211** (9): 1152–4. PMID 9364230.

38. Moll HD, Slone DE, Juzwiak JS, Garrett PD (1987). "Diagonal paramedian approach for removal of ovarian tumors in the mare". *Vet Surg* **16** (6): 456–8. doi:10.1111/j.1532-950X.1987.tb00987.x. PMID 3507181. http://www3.interscience.wiley.com/journal/119849124/abstract.

39. Doran R, Allen D, Gordon B (January 1988). "Use of stapling instruments to aid in the removal of ovarian tumours in mares". *Equine Vet. J.* **20** (1): 37–40. PMID 2835223.

REFERENCES – OVARIAN CYST

1. "Ovarian Cysts Causes, Symptoms, Diagnosis, and Treatment". *eMedicineHealth.com.* http://www.emedicinehealth.com/ovarian_cysts/article_em.htm.

2. http://209.85.165.104/search?q=cache:T1mqp0ojqocJ:medical-dictionary.thefreedictionary.com/hemorrhagic%2Bcyst+Hemorrhagic+cyst&hl=en&ct=clnk&cd=11&gl=us

3. http://209.85.165.104/search?q=cache:QiUSJFPY5GwJ:www.parkermd.com/ovarian-cysts.htm+Hemorrhagic+cyst&hl=en&ct=clnk&cd=9&gl=us

4. Swire MN, Castro-Aragon I, Levine D (2004). "Various sonographic appearances of the hemorrhagic corpus luteum cyst". *Ultrasound Q* **20** (2): 45–58. doi:10.1097/00013644-200406000-00003. PMID 15480190. http://meta.wkhealth.com/pt/pt-core/template-journal/lwwgateway/media/landingpage.htm?issn=0894-8771&volume=20&issue=2&spage=45.

5. [1]

6. *Ovarian Cysts* at eMedicine

7. http://209.85.165.104/search?q=cache:KLaiiA7P8ugJ:health.ivillage.com/gyno/cysts/0,,4ltl,00.html+Hemorrhagic+cyst&hl=en&ct=clnk&cd=8&gl=us

8. *Ovarian Cysts* at eMedicine

9. "Ovarian cysts: Symptoms". *MayoClinic.com.* http://www.mayoclinic.com/health/ovarian-cysts/DS00129/DSECTION=2.

10. [2]

11. "Ovarian Cysts Causes, Symptoms, Diagnosis, and Treatment". *eMedicineHealth.com.* http://www.emedicinehealth.com/ovarian_cysts/page3_em.htm.

12. "Ovarian Cysts - Symptoms, Treatment and Prevention". *HealthScout.* http://www.healthscout.com/ency/1/725/main.html#SymptomsofOvarianCysts.

13. "Ovarian Cysts". http://www.medicineonline.com/topics/O/2/Ovarian-Cysts.html.

14. http://www.nhs.uk/Conditions/Ovarian-cyst/Pages/Symptoms.aspx

15. "Ovarian Cysts Treatment & Monitoring". *Medicine Online.* http://www.medicineonline.com/topics/O/2/Ovarian-Cysts/info/Treatment-&-Monitoring.html.

16. [3]

17. [4]

18. MedlinePlus Encyclopedia CA-125

19. "HealthHints: Gynecologic Health (January/February, 2003)". *Texas AgriLife Extension Service: HealthHints.* http://fcs.tamu.edu/health/health_education_rural_outreach/Health_Hints/2003/jan-feb/gynecologic_health.php.

20. http://ovariancystinfo.weebly.com Cyst on Ovary

REFERENCES – GERM CELL TUMOR

1. Ulbright TM (2005). "Germ cell tumors of the gonads: review emphasizing problems in differential diagnosis, newly appreciated, and controversial issues". *Mod. Pathol.* **18 Suppl 2:** S61–79. doi:10.1038/modpathol.3800310. PMID 15761467. PubMed **free full text**

2. "eMedicine - Germinoma, Central Nervous System : Article by Daniel D Mais, MD". http://www.emedicine.com/med/topic2246.htm. Retrieved on 2007-11-03.

3. Robbins, Basic Pathology; ISBN 0-7216-9274-5, 7th edition, pg 664.

4. MESH 2008: Teratocarcinoma

5. Mediastinal germ cell tumor in a child with precocious puberty and Klinefelter syndrome. Gregory G. Bebb, Frederic W. Grannis, Jr, Isaac B. Paz, Marilyn L. Slovak, Robert Chilcote. Ann Thorac Surg 1998;66:547-548. Abstract

6. International Germ Cell Consensus Classification: a prognostic factor-based staging system for metastatic germ cell cancers. International Germ Cell Cancer Collaborative Group. J Clin Oncol. 1997 Feb;15(2):594-603 PubMed abstract

7. Stankovic ZB, Djukic MK, Savic D, Lukac BJ, Djuricic S, Sedlecki K, Zdravkovic D (2006). "Pre-operative differentiation of pediatric ovarian tumors: morphological scoring system and tumor markers". *J. Pediatr. Endocrinol. Metab.* **19** (10): 1231–8. PMID 17172084.

8. CureSearch.org press release re Germ Cell Cancer

REFERENCES – DESMOPLASTIC SMALL ROUND CELL TUMOR

1. Lee YS, Hsiao CH (October 2007). "Desmoplastic small round cell tumor: a clinicopathologic, immunohistochemical and molecular study of four patients". *J. Formos. Med. Assoc.* **106** (10): 854–60. doi:10.1016/S0929-6646(08)60051-0. PMID 17964965. http://ajws.elsevier.com/ajws_pubmed/pubmed_switch.asp?journal_issn=0929-6646&art_pub_year=2007&art_pub_month=10&art_pub_vol=106&art_sp=854.

2. Bland AE, Shah AA, Piscitelli JT, Bentley RC, Secord AA (2007). "Desmoplastic small round cell tumor masquerading as advanced ovarian cancer". *Int J Gynecol Cancer* **18**: 847. doi:10.1111/j.1525-1438.2007.01110.x. PMID 18081791.

3. Murphy AJ, Bishop K, Pereira C, et al. (December 2008). "A new molecular variant of desmoplastic small round cell tumor: significance of WT1 immunostaining in this entity". *Hum. Pathol.* **39** (12): 1763–70. doi:10.1016/j.humpath.2008.04.019. PMID 18703217. http://linkinghub.elsevier.com/retrieve/pii/S0046-8177(08)00222-0.

4. Gerald WL, Haber DA (June 2005). "The EWS-WT1 gene fusion in desmoplastic small round cell tumor". *Semin. Cancer Biol.* **15** (3): 197–205. doi:10.1016/j.semcancer.2005.01.005. PMID 15826834. http://linkinghub.elsevier.com/retrieve/pii/S1044-579X(05)00006-4.

5. Li H, Smolen GA, Beers LF, et al. (2008). "Adenosine transporter ENT4 is a direct target of EWS/WT1 translocation product and is highly expressed in desmoplastic small round cell tumor". *PLoS ONE* **3** (6): e2353. doi:10.1371/journal.pone.0002353. PMID 18523561. PMC: 2394657. http://www.plosone.org/article/info:doi/10.1371/journal.pone.0002353.

6. Farmer KCR, Hawley PR, Phillips RKS: Desmoid disease. In: Phillips RKS, Spigelman AD, Thomson JPS, et al. ed. Familial Adenomatous Polyposis and Other Polyposis Syndromes, Boston: Little, Brown; 1994

7. Talarico F, Iusco D, Negri L, Belinelli D (2007). "Combined resection and multi-agent adjuvant chemotherapy for intra-abdominal desmoplastic small round cell tumour: case report and review of the literature". *G Chir* **28** (10): 367–70. PMID 17915050. http://www.giornalechirurgia.it/index.php?PAGE=article&ID=2393.

8. Aguilera D, Hayes-Jordan A, Anderson P, Woo S, Pearson M, Green H (2008). "Outpatient and home chemotherapy with novel local control strategies in desmoplastic small round cell tumor". *Sarcoma* **2008:** 261589. doi:10.1155/2008/261589. PMID 18566684.

9. Official website for Stehlin Foundation

REFERENCES – SURFACE EPITHELIAL STROMAL TUMOR

1. Cotran, Ramzi S.; Kumar, Vinay; Fausto, Nelson; Nelso Fausto; Robbins, Stanley L.; Abbas, Abul K. (2005). *Robbins and Cotran pathologic basis of disease* (7th ed.). St. Louis, Mo: Elsevier Saunders. ISBN 0-7216-0187-1.

2. NCI Issues Clinical Announcement for Preferred Method of Treatment for Advanced Ovarian Cancer, January 2006

REFERENCES – SEX CORD GONADAL STROMAL TUMOR

1. Sajadi KP, Dalton RR, Brown JA (2009). "Sex cord-gonadal stromal tumor of the rete testis". *Adv Urol*: 624173. doi:10.1155/2009/624173. PMID 19125206.

2. Chivukula M, Hunt J, Carter G, Kelley J, Patel M, Kanbour-Shakir A (January 2007). "Recurrent gynandroblastoma of ovary-A case report: a molecular and immunohistochemical analysis". *Int. J. Gynecol. Pathol.* **26** (1): 30–3. doi:10.1097/01.pgp.0000225387.48868.39. PMID 17197894. http://meta.wkhealth.com/pt/pt-core/template-journal/lwwgateway/media/landingpage.htm?an=00004347-200701000-00006.

3. Limaïem F, Lahmar A, Ben Fadhel C, Bouraoui S, M'zabi-Regaya S (February 2008). "Gynandroblastoma. Report of an unusual ovarian tumour and literature review". *Pathologica* **100** (1): 13–7. PMID 18686520.

4. Broshears JR, Roth LM (October 1997). "Gynandroblastoma with elements resembling juvenile granulosa cell tumor". *Int. J. Gynecol. Pathol.* **16** (4): 387–91. PMID 9421080.

5. Antunes L, Ounnoughene-Piet M, Hennequin V, Maury F, Lemelle JL, Labouyrie E, Plénat F (April 2002). "Gynandroblastoma of the testis in an infant: a morphological, immunohistochemical and in-situ hybridization report". *Histopathology* **40** (4): 395–7. PMID 11943029. http://www3.interscience.wiley.com/resolve/openurl?genre=article&sid=nlm:pubmed&issn=0309-0167&date=2002&volume=40&issue=4&spage=395.

6. Schneider DT, Jänig U, Calaminus G, Göbel U, Harms D (October 2003). "Ovarian sex cord-stromal tumors--a clinicopathological study of 72 cases from the Kiel Pediatric Tumor Registry". *Virchows Arch.* **443** (4): 549–60. doi:10.1007/s00428-003-0869-0. PMID 12910419. http://dx.doi.org/10.1007/s00428-003-0869-0.

7. McCluggage WG, McKenna M, McBride HA (2007). "CD56 is a sensitive and diagnostically useful immunohistochemical marker of ovarian sex cord-stromal tumors". *Int. J. Gynecol. Pathol.* **26** (3): 322–7. doi:10.1097/01.pgp.0000236947.59463.87. PMID 17581419.

8. Deavers MT, Malpica A, Liu J, Broaddus R, Silva EG (June 2003). "Ovarian sex cord-stromal tumors: an immunohistochemical study including a comparison of calretinin and inhibin". *Mod. Pathol.* **16** (6): 584–90. doi:10.1097/01.MP.0000073133.79591.A1. PMID 12808064. http://dx.doi.org/10.1097/01.MP.0000073133.79591.A1.

9. Takeuchi M, Matsuzaki K, Sano N, Furumoto H, Nishitani H (2008). "Ovarian fibromatosis: magnetic resonance imaging findings with pathologic correlation". *J Comput Assist Tomogr* **32** (5): 776–7. doi:10.1097/RCT.0b013e318157689a. PMID 18830110. http://meta.wkhealth.com/pt/ptcore/template-journal/lwwgateway/media/landingpage.htm?an=00004728-200809000-00018.

10. Kitajima K, Kaji Y, Sugimura K (2008). "Usual and unusual MRI findings of ovarian fibroma: correlation with pathologic findings". *Magn Reson Med Sci* **7** (1): 43–8. PMID 18460848. http://joi.jlc.jst.go.jp/JST.JSTAGE/mrms/7.43?from=PubMed.

11. Chan JK, Zhang M, Kaleb V, Loizzi V, Benjamin J, Vasilev S, Osann K, Disaia PJ (January 2005). "Prognostic factors responsible for survival in sex cord stromal tumors of the ovary--a multivariate analysis". *Gynecol. Oncol.* **96** (1): 204–9. doi:10.1016/j.ygyno.2004.09.019. PMID 15589602. http://linkinghub.elsevier.com/retrieve/pii/S0090-8258(04)00743-7.

12. Schneider DT, Calaminus G, Harms D, Göbel U (June 2005). "Ovarian sex cord-stromal tumors in children and adolescents". *J Reprod Med* **50** (6): 439–46. PMID 16050568

REFERENCES – FOLLICULAR CYST OF OVARY

1. "Follicular cyst of the ovary definition". *MedTerms*. http://www.medterms. com/script/main/art.asp?articlekey=8442.

2. "Ovarian Cysts". *The Institute for Female Alternative Medicine.*. http://www. alternativesurgery.com/education/ovariancysts.php.

3. [1]

4. [2]

5. "Ovarian cysts". *Mayo Clinic*. http://www.mayoclinic.com/health/ovarian-cysts/DS00129.

6. http://209.85.165.104/search?q=cache:nJwAOrHyWhIJ:www.usc.edu/hsc/dental/opath/Chapters/DictionaryF.html+%22follicular+cyst%22&hl=en&ct=clnk&cd=35&gl=us

REFERENCES – BRENNER TUMOR

1. Marwah N, Mathur SK, Marwah S, Singh S, Karwasra RK, Arora B (2005). "Malignant Brenner tumour--a case report". *Indian J Pathol Microbiol* **48** (2): 251–2. PMID 16758686.

2. Green GE, Mortele KJ, Glickman JN, Benson CB (2006). "Brenner tumors of the ovary: sonographic and computed tomographic imaging features". *J Ultrasound Med* **25** (10): 1245–51; quiz 1252–4. PMID 16998096. http://www.jultrasoundmed.org/cgi/pmidlookup?view=long&pmid=16998096.

3. Caccamo D, Socias M, Truchet C (1991). "Malignant Brenner tumor of the testis and epididymis". *Arch. Pathol. Lab. Med.* **115** (5): 524–7. PMID 2021324.

4. Lamping JD, Blythe JG (1977). "Bilateral Brenner tumors: a case report and review of the literature". *Hum. Pathol.* **8** (5): 583–5. doi:10.1016/S0046-8177(77)80117-2. PMID 903146.

5. Philipp, Elliot Elias; O'Dowd, Michael J. (2000). *The history of obstetrics and gynaecology*. Carnforth, Lancs: Parthenon. p. 586. ISBN 1-85070-040-0.

REFERENCES – KRUKENBERG TUMOR

1. Rosai J. Rosai and Ackerman's Surgical Pathology. Vol 2, p1708, 2004

2. *doctor/620* at Who Named It?

3. F. E. Krukenberg: Über das Fibrosarcoma ovarii mucocellulare (carcinomatodes). Archiv für Gynäkologie, Berlin, 1896, 50: 287-321.

4. Rosai J. Rosai and Ackerman's Surgical Pathology. Vol 2, p1708, 2004

REFERENCES – PRIMARY PERITONEAL CANCER

1. Jaaback KS, Ludeman L, Clayton NL, Hirschowitz L (2006). "Primary peritoneal carcinoma in a UK cancer center: comparison with advanced ovarian carcinoma over a 5-year period". *Int. J. Gynecol. Cancer* **16 Suppl 1:** 123–8. doi:10.1111/j.1525-1438.2006.00474.x. PMID 16515579.

2. "Gynecologic Cancer Treatment — Primary Peritoneal Cancer — Dana-Farber Cancer Institute". http://www.dfci.harvard.edu/pat/adult/gynecologic-cancer/diseases-treated/primary-peritoneal-cancer.html.

3. Burger RA, Sill MW, Monk BJ, Greer BE, Sorosky JI (November 2007). "Phase II trial of bevacizumab in persistent or recurrent epithelial ovarian cancer or primary peritoneal cancer: a Gynecologic Oncology Group Study". *J. Clin. Oncol.* **25** (33): 5165–71. doi:10.1200/JCO.2007.11.5345. PMID 18024863. http://www.jco.org/cgi/pmidlookup?view=long&pmid=18024863.

4. "New Drug Combination for Ovarian and Primary Peritoneal Cancers - National Cancer Institute". http://www.cancer.gov/clinicaltrials/ft-MAYO-MC0261.

5. "eMedicine — Peritoneal Cancer : Article by Wissam Bleibel". http://www.emedicine.com/med/TOPIC1795.HTM.

6. Alphs HH, Zahurak ML, Bristow RE, Díaz-Montes TP (December 2006). "Predictors of surgical outcome and survival among elderly women diagnosed with ovarian and primary peritoneal cancer". *Gynecol. Oncol.* **103** (3): 1048–53. doi:10.1016/j.ygyno.2006.06.019. PMID 16876237. http://linkinghub.elsevier.com/retrieve/pii/S0090-8258(06)00505-1.

HEALTHSCOUTER

GNU FREE DOCUMENTATION LICENSE

0. PREAMBLE

The purpose of this License is to make a manual, textbook, or other functional and useful document "free" in the sense of freedom: to assure everyone the effective freedom to copy and redistribute it, with or without modifying it, either commercially or noncommercially. Secondarily, this License preserves for the author and publisher a way to get credit for their work, while not being considered responsible for modifications made by others.

This License is a kind of "copyleft", which means that derivative works of the document must themselves be free in the same sense. It complements the GNU General Public License, which is a copyleft license designed for free software.

We have designed this License in order to use it for manuals for free software, because free software needs free documentation: a free program should come with manuals providing the same freedoms that the software does. But this License is not limited to software manuals; it can be used for any textual work, regardless of subject matter or whether it is published as a printed book. We recommend this License principally for works whose purpose is instruction or reference.

1. APPLICABILITY AND DEFINITIONS

This License applies to any manual or other work, in any medium, that contains a notice placed by the copyright holder saying it can be distributed under the terms of this License. Such a notice grants a world-wide, royalty-free license, unlimited in duration, to use that work under the conditions stated herein. The "Document", herein, refers to any such manual or work. Any member of the public is a licensee, and is addressed as "you". You accept the license if you copy, modify or distribute the work in a way requiring permission under copyright law.

A "Modified Version" of the Document means any work containing the Document or a portion of it, either copied verbatim, or with modifications and/or translated into another language.

A "Secondary Section" is a named appendix or a front-matter section of the Document that deals exclusively with the relationship of the publishers or authors of the Document to the Document's overall subject (or to related matters) and contains nothing that could fall directly within that overall subject. (Thus, if the Document is in part a textbook of mathematics, a Secondary Section may not explain any mathematics.) The relationship could be a matter of historical connection with the subject or with related matters, or of legal, commercial, philosophical, ethical or political position regarding them.

The "Invariant Sections" are certain Secondary Sections whose titles are designated, as being those of Invariant Sections, in the notice that says that the Document is released under this License. If a section does not fit the above definition of Secondary then it is not allowed to be designated as Invariant. The Document may contain zero Invariant Sections. If the Document does not identify any Invariant Sections then there are none.

The "Cover Texts" are certain short passages of text that are listed, as Front-Cover Texts or Back-Cover Texts, in the notice that says that the Document is released under this License. A Front-Cover Text may be at most 5 words, and a Back-Cover Text may be at most 25 words.

A "Transparent" copy of the Document means a machine-readable copy, represented in a format whose specification is available to the general public, that is suitable for revising the document straightforwardly with generic text editors or (for images composed of pixels) generic paint programs or (for drawings) some widely available drawing editor, and that is suitable for input to text formatters or for automatic translation to a variety of formats suitable for input to text formatters. A copy made in an otherwise Transparent file format whose markup, or absence of markup, has been arranged to thwart or discourage subsequent modification by readers is not Transparent. An image format is not Transparent if used for any substantial amount of text. A copy that is not "Transparent" is called "Opaque".

Examples of suitable formats for Transparent copies include plain ASCII without markup, Texinfo input format, LaTeX input format, SGML or XML using a publicly available DTD, and standard-conforming simple HTML, PostScript or PDF designed for human modification. Examples of transparent image formats include PNG, XCF and JPG. Opaque formats include proprietary formats that can be read and edited only by proprietary word processors, SGML or XML for which the DTD and/or processing tools are not generally available, and the machine-generated HTML, PostScript or PDF produced by some word processors for output purposes only.

The "Title Page" means, for a printed book, the title page itself, plus such following pages as are needed to hold, legibly, the material this License requires to appear in the title page. For works in formats which do not have any title page as such, "Title Page" means the text near the most prominent appearance of the work's title, preceding the beginning of the body of the text.

A section "Entitled XYZ" means a named subunit of the Document whose title either is precisely XYZ or contains XYZ in parentheses following text that translates XYZ in another language. (Here XYZ stands for a specific section name mentioned below, such as "Acknowledgements", "Dedications", "Endorsements", or "History".) To "Preserve the Title" of such a section when you modify the Document means that it remains a section "Entitled XYZ" according to this definition.

The Document may include Warranty Disclaimers next to the notice which states that this License applies to the Document. These Warranty Disclaimers are considered to be included by reference in this License, but only as regards disclaiming warranties: any other implication that these Warranty Disclaimers may have is void and has no effect on the meaning of this License.

2. VERBATIM COPYING

You may copy and distribute the Document in any medium, either commercially or noncommercially, provided that this License, the copyright notices, and the license notice saying this License applies to the Document are reproduced in all copies, and that you add no other conditions whatsoever to those of this License. You may not use technical measures to obstruct or control the reading or further copying of the copies you make or distribute. However, you may accept compensation in exchange for copies. If you distribute a large enough number of copies you must also follow the conditions in section 3.

You may also lend copies, under the same conditions stated above, and you may publicly display copies.

3. COPYING IN QUANTITY

If you publish printed copies (or copies in media that commonly have printed covers) of the Document, numbering more than 100, and the Document's license notice requires Cover Texts, you must enclose the copies in covers that carry, clearly and legibly, all these Cover Texts: Front-Cover Texts on the front cover, and Back-Cover Texts on the back cover. Both covers must also clearly and legibly identify you as the publisher of these copies. The front cover must present the full title with all words of the title equally prominent and visible. You may add other material on the covers in addition. Copying with changes limited to the covers, as long as they preserve the title of the Document and satisfy these conditions, can be treated as verbatim copying in other respects.

If the required texts for either cover are too voluminous to fit legibly, you should put the first ones listed (as many as fit reasonably) on the actual cover, and continue the rest onto adjacent pages.

If you publish or distribute Opaque copies of the Document numbering more than 100, you must either include a machine-readable Transparent copy along with each Opaque copy, or state in or with each Opaque copy a computer-network location from which the general network-using public has access to download using public-standard network protocols a complete Transparent copy of the Document, free of added material. If you use the latter option, you must take reasonably prudent steps, when you begin distribution of Opaque copies in quantity, to ensure that this Transparent copy will remain thus accessible at the stated location until at least one year after the last time you distribute an Opaque copy (directly or through your agents or retailers) of that edition to the public.

It is requested, but not required, that you contact the authors of the Document well before redistributing any large number of copies, to give them a chance to provide you with an updated version of the Document.

4. MODIFICATIONS

You may copy and distribute a Modified Version of the Document under the conditions of sections 2 and 3 above, provided that you release the Modified Version under precisely this License, with the Modified Version filling the role of the Document, thus licensing distribution and modification of the Modified Version to whoever possesses a copy of it. In addition, you must do these things in the Modified Version:

A. Use in the Title Page (and on the covers, if any) a title distinct from that of the Document, and from those of previous versions (which should, if there were any, be listed in the History section of the Document). You may use the same title as a previous version if the original publisher of that version gives permission.

B. List on the Title Page, as authors, one or more persons or entities responsible for authorship of the modifications in the Modified Version, together with at least five of the principal authors of the Document (all of its principal authors, if it has fewer than five), unless they release you from this requirement.

C. State on the Title page the name of the publisher of the Modified Version, as the publisher.

D. Preserve all the copyright notices of the Document.

E. Add an appropriate copyright notice for your modifications adjacent to the other copyright notices.

F. Include, immediately after the copyright notices, a license notice giving the public permission to use the Modified Version under the terms of this License, in the form shown in the Addendum below.

G. Preserve in that license notice the full lists of Invariant Sections and required Cover Texts given in the Document's license notice.

H. Include an unaltered copy of this License.

I. Preserve the section Entitled "History", Preserve its Title, and add to it an item stating at least the title, year, new authors, and publisher of the Modified Version as given on the Title Page. If there is no section Entitled "History" in the Document, create one stating the title, year, authors, and publisher of the Document as given on its Title Page, then add an item describing the Modified Version as stated in the previous sentence.

J. Preserve the network location, if any, given in the Document for public access to a Transparent copy of the Document, and likewise the network locations given in the Document for previous versions it was based on. These may be placed in the "History" section. You may omit a network location for a work that was published at least four years before the Document itself, or if the original publisher of the version it refers to gives permission.

K. For any section entitled "Acknowledgements" or "Dedications", Preserve the Title of the section, and preserve in the section all the substance and tone of each of the contributor acknowledgements and/or dedications given therein.

L. Preserve all the Invariant Sections of the Document, unaltered in their text and in their titles. Section numbers or the equivalent are not considered part of the section titles.

M. Delete any section entitled "Endorsements". Such a section may not be included in the Modified Version.

N. Do not retitle any existing section to be entitled "Endorsements" or to conflict in title with any Invariant Section.

O. Preserve any Warranty Disclaimers.

If the Modified Version includes new front-matter sections or appendices that qualify as Secondary Sections and contain no material copied from the Document, you may at your option designate some or all of these sections as Invariant. To do this, add their titles to the list of Invariant Sections in the Modified Version's license notice. These titles must be distinct from any other section titles.

You may add a section entitled "Endorsements", provided it contains nothing but endorsements of your Modified Version by various parties—for example, statements of peer review or that the text has been approved by an organization as the authoritative definition of a standard.

You may add a passage of up to five words as a Front-Cover Text, and a passage of up to 25 words as a Back-Cover Text, to the end of the list of Cover Texts in the Modified Version. Only one passage of Front-Cover Text and one of Back-Cover Text may be added by (or through arrangements made by) any one entity. If the Document already includes a Cover Text for the same cover, previously added by you or by arrangement made by the same entity you are acting on behalf of, you may not add another; but you may replace the old one, on explicit permission from the previous publisher that added the old one.

The author(s) and publisher(s) of the Document do not by this License give permission to use their names for publicity for or to assert or imply endorsement of any Modified Version.

5. COMBINING DOCUMENTS

You may combine the Document with other documents released under this License, under the terms defined in section 4 above for modified versions, provided that you include in the combination all of the Invariant Sections of all of the original documents, unmodified, and list them all as Invariant Sections of your combined work in its license notice, and that you preserve all their Warranty Disclaimers.

The combined work need only contain one copy of this License, and multiple identical Invariant Sections may be replaced with a single copy. If there are multiple Invariant Sections with the same name but different contents, make the title of each such section unique by adding at the end of it, in parentheses, the name of the original author or publisher of that section if known, or else a unique number. Make the same adjustment to the section titles in the list of Invariant Sections in the license notice of the combined work.

In the combination, you must combine any sections entitled "History" in the various original documents, forming one section entitled "History";

likewise combine any sections entitled "Acknowledgements", and any sections entitled "Dedications". You must delete all sections entitled "Endorsements."

6. COLLECTIONS OF DOCUMENTS

You may make a collection consisting of the Document and other documents released under this License, and replace the individual copies of this License in the various documents with a single copy that is included in the collection, provided that you follow the rules of this License for verbatim copying of each of the documents in all other respects.

You may extract a single document from such a collection, and distribute it individually under this License, provided you insert a copy of this License into the extracted document, and follow this License in all other respects regarding verbatim copying of that document.

7. AGGREGATION WITH INDEPENDENT WORKS

A compilation of the Document or its derivatives with other separate and independent documents or works, in or on a volume of a storage or distribution medium, is called an "aggregate" if the copyright resulting from the compilation is not used to limit the legal rights of the compilation's users beyond what the individual works permit. When the Document is included in an aggregate, this License does not apply to the other works in the aggregate which are not themselves derivative works of the Document.

If the Cover Text requirement of section 3 is applicable to these copies of the Document, then if the Document is less than one half of the entire aggregate, the Document's Cover Texts may be placed on covers that bracket the Document within the aggregate, or the electronic equivalent of covers if the Document is in electronic form. Otherwise they must appear on printed covers that bracket the whole aggregate.

8. TRANSLATION

Translation is considered a kind of modification, so you may distribute translations of the Document under the terms of section 4. Replacing Invariant Sections with translations requires special permission from their copyright holders, but you may include translations of some or all Invariant Sections in addition to the original versions of these Invariant Sections. You may include a translation of this License, and all the license notices in the Document, and any Warranty Disclaimers, provided that you also include the original English version of this License and the original versions of those notices and disclaimers. In case of a disagreement between the translation and the original version of this License or a notice or disclaimer, the original version will prevail.

If a section in the Document is entitled "Acknowledgements", "Dedications", or "History", the requirement (section 4) to Preserve its Title (section 1) will typically require changing the actual title.

9. TERMINATION

You may not copy, modify, sublicense, or distribute the Document except as expressly provided for under this License. Any other attempt to copy, modify, sublicense or distribute the Document is void, and will automatically terminate your rights under this License. However, parties who have received copies, or rights, from you under this License will not have their licenses terminated so long as such parties remain in full compliance.

10. FUTURE REVISIONS OF THIS LICENSE

The Free Software Foundation may publish new, revised versions of the GNU Free Documentation License from time to time. Such new versions will be similar in spirit to the present version, but may differ in detail to address new problems or concerns. See http://www.gnu.org/copyleft/.

Each version of the License is given a distinguishing version number. If the Document specifies that a particular numbered version of this License "or any later version" applies to it, you have the option of following the terms and conditions either of that specified version or of any later version that has been published (not as a draft) by the Free Software Foundation. If the Document does not specify a version number of this License, you may choose any version ever published (not as a draft) by the Free Software Foundation.

INDEX

www.ingramcontent.com/pod-product-compliance
Lightning Source LLC
Chambersburg PA
CBHW070801290326
41931CB00011BA/2102